Understanding the Nursing Process

Understanding the Nursing Process

THIRD EDITION

Leslie D. Atkinson, R.N., M.S.
Instructor, Nursing Program
Normandale Community College
Bloomington, Minnesota

Mary Ellen Murray, R.N., M.S.
Assistant Professor
Raymond Walters College
University of Cincinnati
Cincinnati, Ohio

Illustrated by Mark Atkinson

Macmillan Publishing Company
NEW YORK

Collier Macmillan Canada, Inc.
TORONTO

Collier Macmillan Publishers
LONDON

Earlier edition(s), entitled UNDERSTANDING THE NURSING PROCESS by Leslie D. Atkinson and Mary Ellen Murray copyright © 1980 and 1983 by Macmillan Publishing Co., Inc.

Macmillan Publishing Company
866 Third Avenue, New York, New York 10022

Collier Macmillan Canada, Inc.
Collier Macmillan Publishers • London

Library of Congress Cataloging in Publication Data

Atkinson, Leslie D.
  Understanding the nursing process.

  Bibliography: p.
  Includes index.
  1. Nursing. 2. Diagnosis. I. Murray, Mary Ellen.
II. Title. [DNLM: 1. Nursing Process. WY 100 A876u]
ISBN 0-02-304520-5

Printing: 1 2 3 4 5 6 7 8   Year: 6 7 8 9 0 1 2 3 4

Dedication
To Gary
To Peter

Preface to the Third Edition

Since the publication of the first edition of *Understanding the Nursing Process* in 1980, we have seen an increasing necessity and responsibility for students to enter the profession of nursing with a consistent and organized framework for approaching patient care. This framework or way of "thinking as a nurse" is best presented and developed very early in the student's educational program, regardless of its length. We feel the nursing process and the concept of care planning should be introduced in the first nursing course, even though the student may not yet have the educational background to understand complex treatments and plans of care. This text is designed to introduce the process, to motivate the student to use the process, and to give the student time to incorporate problem-solving thinking into all aspects of patient care. Because this text is written for a student entering nursing education, terminology and nursing/medical interventions are kept simple and theoretical discussions of nursing, nursing process, and frameworks for nursing are presented only in the very practical sense of application to patient care planning situations.

We continue to see trends within health care that make the nursing process an essential tool in all types of delivery systems:

1. Decreasing length of stay in the hospital. Patients are being discharged from the hospital in less and less time because of limits imposed by health insurance payments. Same-day surgery is a new and popular alternative to hospitalization, further limiting the time the professional nurse has to spend with an individual patient. Assessment and planning become even more crucial as families and home health agencies begin to provide care previously done by nurses in the hospital.

2. Expansion of home health care facilities. Various types of health care personnel such as aides, L.P.N.s, and R.N.s are providing care to people in their homes to facilitate early hospital discharge. Without a thorough assessment and plan developed by the professional nurse, the care

these patients receive at home by various people is unor-
ganized at best and may be doing little to promote wellness
and independence from the system.

3. Continued development of standardized terminology and
    problem areas for nursing diagnoses with increasing na-
    tional acceptance and usage in the clinical setting.
4. Entry into independent practice of professional nurses.
5. Increasing scope of independent nursing actions.
6. Increasing acuity levels of hospitalized patients.
7. Increasing legal accountability of nurses for nursing prac-
    tice.
8. Institutional quality of care standards which require that
    each patient has a documented care plan within 24 hours
    of admission.
9. Institutional policies which require that nursing care plans
    be retained as part of the patient's permanent records.
10. Utilization of the registered nurse licensing examination
    based on the nursing process steps of: assessing, analyzing,
    planning, implementing, and evaluating.

This edition of *Understanding the Nursing Process* will continue
to use a four-step approach to the nursing process: *assessment, planning, implementation*, and *evaluation*. Some texts are using a five-
step approach to the nursing process but without uniformity in desig-
nation of the fifth step. The fifth step of *analysis* is broken out of
assessment and planning as described by the National Council of
State Boards of Nursing for the testing categories on the R.N. licensing exam. The American Nurses' Association's "Nursing—A Social
Policy Statement," c. 1980, elaborates on the activity of *diagnosis*
while continuing to utilize the terms of assessment, planning, implementation, and evaluation as the components of the nursing process.

> The nursing process requires a systematic approach to the *assessment*
> of the patient's situation, which includes reconciliation of patient/
> family and nurse perceptions of the situation; a *plan* for nursing
> actions, which include patient/family participation in goal setting;
> joint *implementation* of the plan; and *evaluation*, which includes
> patient/family participation.

Rather than choose between analysis, nursing diagnosis, and
problem identification as the fifth step, we will retain the clarity of
the four-step division of the nursing process with expansion of analysis as an activity in assessment. We believe that determination of

goals with the patient is an act of synthesis rather than analysis and choose to retain this activity and related content within the planning step of the nursing process. In the introduction to the text, we provide the student with a table comparing the four- and various five-step divisions of the process with the related activities.

As in the second edition, the third edition will emphasize a practical approach to utilizing the nursing process and developing patient care plans. Other features of the third edition include

1. A reading level appropriate to a student entering any school of nursing.
2. Utilization of the approved nursing diagnoses from the Fifth National Conference on Nursing Diagnosis, 1982, and the Sixth National Conference on Nursing Diagnosis, 1984. Throughout the text and in the care plans appearing in the appendix, the accepted nursing diagnoses have been identified and applied to patient case situations.
3. A portable, new Nursing Diagnosis Pocketbook, located in the envelope at the back of this book. The Nursing Diagnosis Pocketbook can be easily removed and carried separately for clinical reference.
4. An updated bibliography.
5. Inclusion of the A.N.A. Standards of Nursing Practice.
6. Utilization of various nursing assessment forms for data collection exemplifying several theoretical frameworks.
7. Expansion and updating of Chapter 1, Assessment, in the areas of analysis and nursing diagnosis.
8. Expansion of Chapter 4, Evaluation, to further explain the concept of evaluation as an ongoing, cyclical review of the nursing process and patient care planning.
9. An introduction designed to help the student understand the process and value its use.
10. Four chapters corresponding to the four steps of the nursing process: assessment, planning, implementation, evaluation.
11. Definitions, illustrations, and practice exercises related to the four steps of the nursing process.
12. Definitions enclosed in boxes that stand out from the body of the text.
13. Application of teaching-learning principles within the care-planning process.

14. An appendix that consists of seven care plans spanning growth and development levels from infancy to old age.
15. A writing style, with illustrations, that is designed to make the book more enjoyable.

We wish to express our appreciation to the nurse educators who have given us encouragement and constructive criticism from our first two editions and ask you to continue to do so. We wish to thank our students who continually force us to apply our theoretical concepts to actual patient care situations in an efficient, effective way. We wish to thank our colleagues at Normandale Community College, Bloomington, Minnesota, and Raymond Walters College, University of Cincinnati, Ohio, for sharing their experiences in teaching the nursing process. We also wish to acknowledge the contributions of Tom Olson as the author of care plan #7 in the appendix and Mark Atkinson for his art work.

Contents

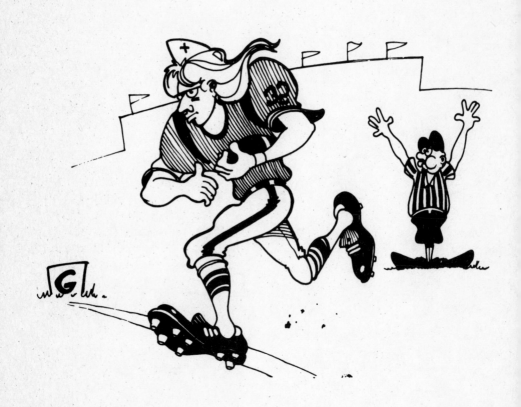

The Nursing Process

THE NURSE WHO SAVED FOOTBALL
(A Totally Untrue Story)

Long ago, there existed a group of people with nothing to do on Sunday afternoons. One of them, John, was a very scholarly individual who had read about a game called football. He decided this game might give him and his friends something to do on those quiet Sundays. He told his friends all about the game and how it was played. Soon they all understood the game very well. They set up the field, erected goalposts, and bought a football. The next Sunday they were all set for some real action (on the field). They divided themselves into two teams and started to play. Now John, the scholarly individual, being the founder of the game, felt he should be the quarterback, since he weighed about 30 pounds less than everyone else and was no fool. Everyone agreed to this arrangement. John called his team into a huddle and said, "Let's get a goal!" So they lined up and started to play. After being sacked 47 times, John began to feel there was something wrong with his game. Football was definitely not a lot of fun for John that day. The next day at practice the team tried to figure out what went wrong. Some blamed John, some blamed the field, some wanted to quit and go back to being bored. One player, who worked as a nurse in a local hospital, said, "I think I have a suggestion. When I give nursing care I use the nursing process to develop a plan of care for my patients. I think our team needs to do the same thing and develop a GAME PLAN." So they did. They wrote a play book and coordinated their efforts to advance the ball. Of course, the next Sunday they creamed their opponents 70 to 3. And that's how the nursing process saved football.

1

NURSING: WHAT IS IT?

Nursing has been described in many different ways by many different leaders and theorists in nursing. What is special about nursing? What service do we provide to our patients that no other health care professional provides? In 1980 the American Nurses' Association, which is the professional organization for nurses in the Untied States, developed a definition that is current and basic to describe the scope of nursing practice.

> Nursing is the diagnosis and treatment of human responses to actual or potential health problems. (A.N.A., "Nursing—A Social Policy Statement," 1980)

This means, for example, that nursing is not responsible for diagnosing and treating cancer; the physician does this. Nursing is primarily responsible for diagnosing and treating a patient's *response* to the cancer and medical treatment, such as inadequate nutrition, nausea, altered self-esteem, anxiety, and pain. Nursing is involved in aspects of the medical treatment as when giving a patient prescribed medication or treatments.

THE NURSING PROCESS: WHAT IS IT?

The nursing process is a problem-solving framework for planning and delivering nursing care to patients and their families.

> The nursing process is:

- a way of thinking as a nurse
- a framework of interrelated activities resulting in competent nursing care
- dynamic and cyclical in nature, requiring repeated review
- a scientific, problem-oriented approach to patient care
- an organized approach to diagnose patients' problematic responses to illness or decreased health and provide treatment

The nursing process is divided into four steps:

1. Assessment
   Let me have a look at that.
   Tell me about it.
   What's the problem?

2. Planning
   What are we going to do about it?
   What is the best strategy?
   What do we want to happen?
3. Implementation
   Move into action.
   Carry out the plan.
   Do it, to it!
4. Evaluation
   Did it work?
   Did we end up where we wanted to?
   Are we done or is there more? What's the problem?

During this process, a written nursing care plan is developed. While the above descriptions are an oversimplification, every nurse already has had much practice in using similar problem-solving techniques, even though the terms of the nursing process itself may be unfamiliar. Consider a high-school chemistry class. Students are asked to observe and examine the properties of different chemicals, and to perform a series of planned experiments utilizing those substances. The student then records and evaluates the results. Hopefully, the student, through the use of this scientific problem-solving process, has discovered the solution to the problem of how certain chemicals react. These steps are essentially the same as those utilized in the nursing process. More familiar is the case of the domestic engineer (uncommonly referred to as a father), who observes the chaos of his 7-year-old's bedroom. After giving the scene an eyeball ASSESSMENT, and palpating the bedcovers for any sign of life, he diagnoses the problem, "This room is an absolute mess!" He then sets forth a PLAN of action. He chooses a goal, "That child isn't going out to play until all his toys are put away." He recruits his son to IMPLEMENT the clean-up, and finally EVALUATES the results. These examples point out that a problem-solving process is not only important to the sciences but is also an integral activity of daily living. Similarly, the applied science of nursing utilizes a logical, systematic problem-solving process to deliver its services. This is called the nursing process. Patients' written care plans are based on application of the nursing process. These care plans serve as a guide for patient care.

An alternate breakdown of the nursing process is a five-step sequence that includes the addition of one of the following activities: analysis, problem identification, or nursing diagnosis. A comparison of the four- and five-step formats for the nursing process is shown in Table 1. This text uses the four-step breakdown of the nursing process but includes explanations of analysis and nursing diagnosis (problem identification) in the chapters on assessment and planning.

WHY IS THE NURSING PROCESS IMPORTANT?

When used as a tool in nursing practice, the nursing process can help ensure quality patient care. Without this systematic way of approaching patient care, omissions and duplications begin to occur. A nursing care plan helps to reduce these problems when it is used as a guide in providing care for a particular patient. Just as a physician formulates medical care plans in treating patients' diseases to ensure consistent, responsible medical management, a nurse utilizes the nursing process to create care plans to ensure consistent and responsible nursing management of patients' problems.

While the primary benefit of utilizing the nursing process is improved patient care, there are also definite advantages for the individ-

Table 1   Comparison of the Four- and Five-Step Nursing Process Formats

Five-Step Format	Four-Step Format	Five-Step Format
1. Assessment	1. Assessment	1. Assessment
2. Nursing Diagnosis (problem identification)	Collect patient data Make nursing diagnoses	
3. Planning	2. Planning Set priorities Select goals of nursing care Plan nursing interventions	2. Analysis
		3. Planning
4. Implementation	3. Implementation Give nursing care based on plan	4. Implementation
5. Evaluation	4. Evaluation Evaluate goal achievement Review nursing process steps and update plan of care	5. Evaluation

ual nurse who becomes skilled in the use of this tool. Consider the following advantages for the nurse (and the student):

1. **Graduation from an Accredited School of Nursing.** The National League for Nursing, which is the organization responsible for accrediting nursing programs, requires students to have a basic competency in the use of the nursing process upon graduation.*

2. **Confidence.** Care plans resulting from the nursing process let the student or the staff nurse know specifically what problem the patient has, what goals are important for the patient, and how and when they might best be accomplished.

3. **Job Satisfaction.** Good care plans can save time, energy, and the frustration that is generated by trial-and-error nursing from staff members and students whose efforts remain uncoordinated. Coordinating a patient's nursing care through a care plan greatly increases the chances of achieving a successful resolution of health problems. The nurse and student should feel a real sense of accomplishment and professional pride when goals in a care plan are met.

4. **Professional Growth.** Care plans provide an opportunity to share knowledge and experience. Collaboration with colleagues in formulating a nursing care plan will add to an inexperienced nurse's clinical skills. Later, during the process of evaluation, the nurse or student receives the feedback necessary to decide how effective the nursing care plan was in dealing with the patient's problems. If the plan worked well, the nurse may use a similar approach in the future. If it failed, the nurse can explore possible reasons for the undesirable results with the patient, other staff, other students, an instructor, or a clinical nurse specialist.

5. **Aid in Staff Assignments.** Care plans assist charge nurses, team leaders, and nursing instructors in making the most appropriate patient assignments by showing the degree of complexity involved in an individual patient's care plan. Could an aide follow the care plan and provide good care, or is a professional nurse required? Could students work with this patient or is the plan of care beyond their knowledge and experience?

6. **Employment in a Nationally Accredited Hospital.** Hospitals are approved by a national commission to help ensure that pa-

*NLN: *Competencies of the Associate Degree Nurse on Entry into Practice*, Publ. No. 23-1731; c. 1978; New York.

tients receive quality care. The following statement is taken directly from the accreditation manual for hospitals and is a requirement for accreditation. (JCAH, *Accreditation Manual*, 1985).

Standard IV
Individualized, goal-directed nursing care shall be provided to patients through the use of the nursing process.

Interpretation
The nursing process (assessment, planning, intervention, evaluation) shall be documented for each hospitalized patient from admission through discharge. Each patient's nursing needs shall be assessed by a registered nurse at the time of admission or within the period established by nursing department/service policy. These assessment data shall be consistent with the medical plan of care and shall be available to all nursing personnel involved in the care of the patient.

7. **Meeting Standards of Nursing Practice.** The American Nurses' Association has identified eight standards of nursing practice that are activities in the nursing process (A.N.A., *Standards of Nursing Practice*, 1973). See Table 2.

Table 2   Standards of Nursing Practice

   I. The collection of data about the health status of the client/patient is systematic and continuous. The data are accessible, communicated, and recorded.
  II. Nursing diagnoses are derived from health status data.
 III. The plan of nursing care includes goals derived from the nursing diagnoses.
  IV. The plan of nursing care includes the priorities and the prescribed nursing approaches or measures to achieve the goals derived from the nursing diagnoses.
   V. Nursing actions provide for client/patient participation and health promotion, maintenance, and restoration.
  VI. Nursing actions assist the client/patient to maximize his health capabilities.
 VII. The client's/patient's progress or lack of progress toward goal achievement is determined by the client/patient and the nurse.
VIII. The client's/patient's progress or lack of progress toward goal achievement directs reassessment, reordering of priorities, new goal setting, and revision of the plan of nursing care.

Reproduced with the permission of A.N.A. from *Standards of Nursing Practice*, A.N.A., 1973.

There are also advantages for the patient.

1. Participation in Own Care. If patients are able to help formulate their own care plans with the nurse, they gain a sense of their own ability to solve problems. When patients are active participants in their care, they are more likely to be committed to the goals in their care plans and thus achieve improved health.

2. Continuity of Care. The frustration of repeating the same information to each nurse caring for them is greatly reduced. Worries, concerns, and problems need not be communicated to each nurse to ensure that they are handled the way patients want them to be handled. The care plan communicates this information.

3. Improved Quality of Care. Use of the nursing process results in a thorough assessment of the patient at the time of admission. Problems are identified at this time by an R.N., who then develops a plan of nursing care with the patient. This plan, developed by the nurse most familiar with the patient, serves as a guide for other nurses, assistants, and students to follow in providing 24-hour care to the patient. Continuous evaluation and review of the nursing process and plan of care assures a level of care that will better meet changing individual needs. This evaluation is a key part of the nursing process and a patient's written care plan.

Giving nursing care without a care plan is like trying to cook a nameless entree without a recipe. To add to your troubles, you have to share the work for preparing this entree with three other cooks, all in the kitchen at different times. You can all cook, but a plan is needed to tell you what the entree is, how to prepare it, when to serve it, and how the three of you can coordinate your efforts to produce the best entree possible. Similarly, many nurses share in the care of a single patient throughout the 24-hour hospital day. Each nurse is capable of providing care, but a plan is needed to coordinate their efforts.

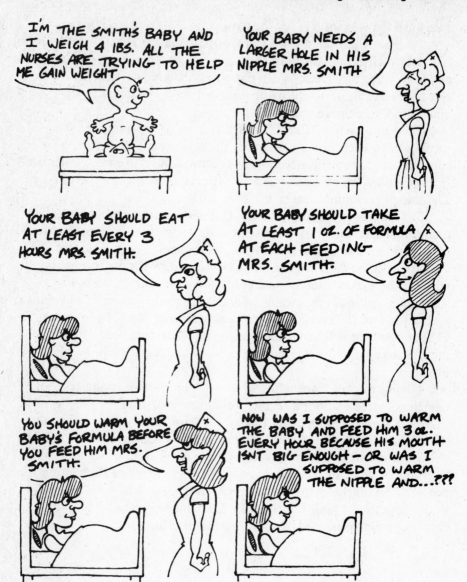

FIGURE I–1. A plan is needed to coordinate the nurse's efforts.

WHAT DOES IT LOOK LIKE?

When the nursing process is being utilized, you will find patients who report that they are receiving excellent nursing care by nurses who really understand their problems and are concerned about them as individuals. You will find an assessment form in the patient's chart indicating that the admitting R.N. took the time to discuss patient and family concerns and current health-related problems. The use of the nursing process will result in a care plan describing the problems and care for each patient. You'll know you've discovered a nursing care plan when, while working in the clinical area, you find a nursing Kardex (by any other name a Kardex is still the same!) with a plan detailing the four elements of care: nursing diagnoses, goals, nursing interventions, and evaluation.

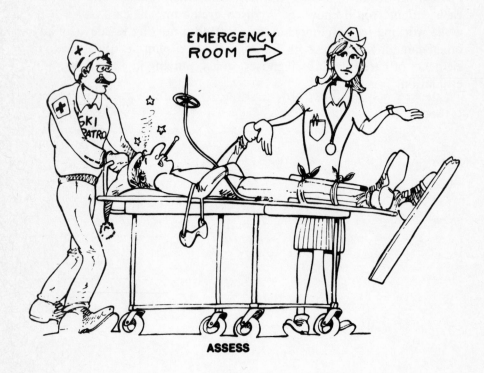

CHAPTER 1

Assessment

Assessment is both the initial step in the nursing process and an ongoing component of every other step in the process. Assessment is a part of each activity the nurse does for and with the patient. Just as the initial nursing assessment is the basis of the patient care plan, so do later assessments contribute to revisions and updates in the care plan as the patient's condition changes. The process of assessment consists of three separate and interdependent activities: data collection, data analysis, and formulating nursing diagnoses.

> **Assessment = Data Collection + Data Analysis + Nursing Diagnosis**

DATA COLLECTION

Because assessment is an ongoing process, there is the potential for the nurse to collect an overwhelming amount of data. It is unrealistic to think that the nurse will record every bit of information that is obtained. One component skill of assessment is the ability to collect *relevant* data. The nursing care plan will be only as good as the data that go into it. A saying used by computerniks nicely illustrates this point, "Garbage in, garbage out."

Data Collection Format

Beginning nursing students are often required to complete nursing data collection assignments. Often these assessments are very lengthy and

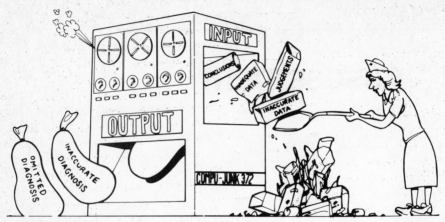

FIGURE 1–1.   Garbage in, garbage out.

time consuming. The purpose of such an assignment is to assist the student in a comprehensive data review and to avoid errors of omission. After the student has demonstrated proficiency in this skill, an abbreviated data collection format similar to those used by staff nurses is recommended. Several examples of such forms will be used throughout this book.

Most health care institutions use a framework to guide the collection of data. The structure of this framework will vary depending on the institution.

One framework that has proven to be helpful is based on the work of psychologist Abraham Maslow, who postulated that all human beings have common basic needs that can be arranged in the following hierarchical order (Table 1–1). Maslow further theorized that basic physical needs must be met to some degree before higher level needs can be met.

The basic physical needs such as food, fluid, and oxygen are considered survival needs and must be met, or at least partially met, if life

Table 1–1

1. Physiological needs—needs that must be met for survival
2. Safety and security needs—things that make the person feel safe and comfortable
3. Love and belonging needs—the need to give and receive love and affection
4. Esteem needs—things that make people feel good about themselves; pride in abilities and accomplishments
5. Self-actualization needs—the need to continue to grow and change; working toward future goals

is to continue. They are the lowest level of needs and usually are satisfied before higher-level needs. Higher-level needs begin with safety/security needs and continue through self-actualization needs.

Using Maslow's theory, consider the following data and the way they are organized.

1. **Physiological needs**
   —temperature 103°F.
   —respirations 36 per minute.
   —liquid stool four times in 1 hour.
   —complains of sharp continuous pain in right lower quadrant.
2. **Safety/security needs**
   —sleeps with night light.
   —mother says 4-year-old Billy is afraid of dark.
   —"My canes slip on the ice so I don't go out much."
3. **Love and belonging**
   —mother and father are with Billy (hospitalized child)
   —"We were married 40 years when my wife died. I miss her so much."
4. **Self-esteem**
   —"I can't even control my bowels—just like a baby."
   —"I just passed the examination for my real estate license."
5. **Self-actualization**
   —"My children are grown with families of their own. Raising them has been my biggest accomplishment."
   —"Teaching nursing students is more than a job. I really feel like I'm contributing to their development and to the profession."

The data recorded within each category may indicate the current status of need satisfaction, alterations in meeting the need, or perhaps interferences in meeting the need. By collecting data in each of these need categories, the nurse develops a format for systematically considering the total patient rather than viewing an illness or a symptom. Comprehensive nursing care results from a consideration of the total patient.

In addition to collecting data using the need levels of Maslow, some consideration of the individual's level of growth and development is necessary. Each chronological age has corresponding developmental tasks, both physical and psychosocial. A developmental task may be thought of as a job, a hurdle, a challenge, or an accomplishment relative to a particular chronological age span. Illness may interfere with

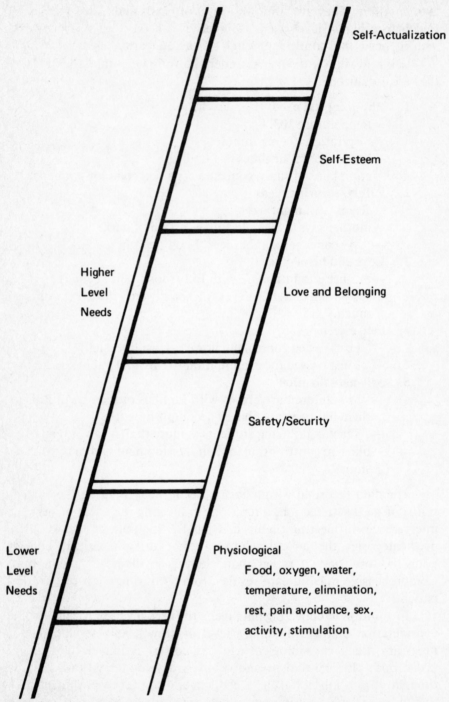

FIGURE 1–2. Maslow's hierarchy of human needs.

completion of developmental tasks appropriate to an age span or with progression to the next developmental level. During illness an individual may even regress to an earlier level of development. For example, the 3-year-old who has been toilet trained for 6 months may begin bed wetting again during hospitalization. The adolescent who has been menstruating for 6 months may cease to menstruate during lengthy confinement in a body cast. Other individuals may appear to arrest at a developmental level during the stress of illness and hospitalization. For example, an infant may fail to begin to crawl and stand during illness. The infant may remain at the developmental level achieved prior to hospitalization and show very little new learning until the stress of hospitalization and illness is reduced. Thus it is important for nurses to assess developmental levels and the tasks associated with each level so they can recognize and understand variations from normal age-related development in patients. By recognizing that a child is regressing to an earlier level or is failing to keep up with peers' development, the nurse may be able to work with the parents and other hospital staff to reduce the damaging influence that hospitalization may have on a child's development. The nurse who has a knowledge of developmental levels and the associated tasks will be able to further individualize patient care. For example, adolescent developmental tasks focus on self-identity. While caring for adolescents, the nurse could choose a nonauthoritative approach which would allow the patient the maximum amount of choice. Similarly, a school-age child's developmental level focuses on independence and project completion. Nursing care that encourages the child to do self-care will promote developmental growth. Table 1-2 is a very brief summary of developmental tasks and the corresponding age spans.

Table 1-2   Major Developmental Tasks

1. Infancy—1 year
   —developing a sense of trust and belonging from relationship with mother and father
   —differentiating self from environment
   —learning to eat solid foods, to walk, to explore, to communicate
2. Toddler—1-3 years
   —developing willpower, independence
   —learning to feed self, to run, communicate verbally, control elimination
   —exploring environment
3. Preschool—3-6 years
   —developing sexual identity
   —developing a sense of initiative
   —working on autonomy, dressing self, washing

Table 1-2   Major Developmental Tasks (cont.)

—developing sense of time, space, distance
—developing imagination
—playing cooperatively
4. School age—6–puberty
—developing a sense of industry; planning and working on projects
—learning the skills for survival in the child's culture
—developing modesty
—learning to read, to calculate, to control emotions
—developing neuromuscular coordination
5. Adolescent—12–18 years
—developing physical maturity
—developing autonomy from home and family
—developing self-identity
—coping with body image
—identifying with peer group

Figure 1–3 is an assessment form that uses Maslow's hierarchy of basic needs as an organizing framework.

In comparison, another institution may use the framework developed by nurse-author Virginia Henderson. Henderson described 14 needs, commonly called activities of daily living (ADLs), that a nurse may help the patient to perform:

1. Breathe normally
2. Eat and drink adequately
3. Eliminate body waste
4. Move and maintain desirable posture
5. Sleep and rest
6. Select suitable clothing, dress and undress
7. Maintain body temperature
8. Keep the body clean and well groomed and protect the integument
9. Avoid dangers in the environment and avoid injuring others
10. Communicate with others
11. Worship according to one's faith
12. Work in such a way that there is a sense of accomplishment
13. Play, or participate in various forms of recreation
14. Learn, discover, or satisfy the curiosity that leads to "normal" development and health, and use available health facilities

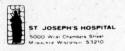

ST JOSEPH'S HOSPITAL
5000 West Chambers Street
Milwaukee Wisconsin 53210

NURSING
HISTORY &
ASSESSMENT

PART A   **(MEDICAL · SURGICAL)**

DATE OF HISTORY	TIME OF HISTORY	INFORMANT(S)

ADMITTING MEDICAL DIAGNOSIS	ARRIVED ON UNIT
	☐ AMBULATORY ☐ WHEELCHAIR ☐ CART ☐ AMBULANCE

REASONS FOR HOSPITALIZATION

HOW HAS THE PATIENT BEEN MANAGING THE ABOVE PROBLEMS AT HOME?

OTHER ILLNESSES OR CONDITIONS (HYPERTENSION, ARTHRITIS, DIABETES, PAST SURGERIES, ETC.)	ALLERGIES (FOOD, MEDICATION, TAPE, DYE, ETC.)

ALCOHOL USAGE	LAST PHYSICIAL EXAM	TYPE OF REACTION

MEDICATION AND DOSAGE PRESCRIBED AND NON-PRESCRIBED	USUAL TIMES TAKEN	TIME OF LAST DOSE	PATIENT'S UNDERSTANDING OF PURPOSE

SUBJECTIVE DATA	OBJECTIVE DATA

COGNITION SENSATION/ COMMUNICATION

LIMITATIONS OR RESTRICTIONS RELATED TO:
VISION: ☐ YES ☐ NO   HEARING: ☐ YES ☐ NO   OTHER: ☐ YES ☐ NO
DESCRIBE:

LAST EYE EXAM

LEVEL OF ORIENTATION (ALERTNESS, ABILITY TO PROCESS INFORMATION, ETC.)

GLASSES _____
CONTACT LENSES _____
ARTIFICIAL EYE _____
HEARING AID _____

APPEARANCE OF EYES, EARS, SPEECH IMPAIRMENTS, ETC.

VENTILATION

REPORT OF DYSPNEA, COUGH, ORTHOPNEA, ETC

HOW MUCH DOES PATIENT SMOKE?

BREATH SOUNDS, SPUTUM, ETC.

RESP. RATE   DEPTH & QUALITY

ST. JOSEPH'S HOSPITAL, MILWAUKEE, WISCONSIN 1982

SIGNATURE _____ R.N.

NURSING HISTORY & ASSESSMENT · PART A

FORM 20441 REV. 5/84

FIGURE 1–3.   Courtesy St. Joseph's Hospital, Milwaukee, Wisconsin.

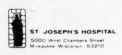

NURSING HISTORY & ASSESSMENT

(MEDICAL-SURGICAL)

PART B

SUBJECTIVE DATA	OBJECTIVE DATA
CIRCULATION	
REPORT OF CHEST PAIN, NUMBNESS, TINGLING, ETC.	PERIPHERAL PULSES, CAPILLARY REFILL, HOMAN'S SIGN, EDEMA, ETC.
	TEMP_____ ☐ O ☐ AX ☐ R PULSES ☐ AP ☐ R_____ QUALITY_____
	BP _____ ☐ R ☐ L ☐ LYING ☐ SITTING ☐ STANDING
NUTRITION / HYDRATION	
REPORTS OF ANOREXIA, NAUSEA, USUAL MEAL PATTERN, ABILITY TO CHEW AND SWALLOW, RECENT CHANGE IN WEIGHT, ETC.	SKIN TURGOR, APPEARANCE OF TONGUE, CONDITION OF TEETH, ETC.
THERAPEUTIC DIET / LAST DENTAL EXAM	HEIGHT / WEIGHT / DENTURES
ELIMINATION	
BOWEL HABITS, VOIDING PATTERN, HEMORRHOIDS, DESCRIPTION OF MENSTRUAL CYCLE, ETC.	DIAPHORESIS, BOWEL SOUNDS, APPEARANCE OF URINE, FECES, VOMITUS, ETC.
REPORTED LBM / LAST PAP SMEAR / LAST PROCTOSCOPIC EXAM	
MOBILITY	
REPORTED INABILITY TO DO ADLS, DIFFICULTY WITH AMBULATION, ETC.	ROM, GAIT, STRENGTH, ENDURANCE, ETC.
	CANE _____ CRUTCHES _____
	WALKER _____ PROSTHESIS _____
INTEGUMENTARY	
REPORTED PRURITIS, ECZEMA, PSORIASIS, ETC.	INSPECTION FOR RASHES, OPEN AREAS, AND ABNORMAL NAIL CONDITION, ETC. NOTE DISTRIBUTION AND QUALITY OF HAIR OR PRESENCE OF WIG
LAST SELF-BREAST EXAM	
COMFORT - REST SLEEP	
REPORT OF PAIN, QUALITY, LOCATION, PRECIPITATING FACTORS, DURATION AND HOW PAIN IS RELIEVED	FACIAL GRIMACING, GUARDING OF AFFECTED AREA, ETC. (NOTE: THERE MAY BE NO OBSERVABLE SIGNS WITH CHRONIC PAIN.)
REPORTED SLEEP PATTERNS AND BEDTIME RITUALS	
PSYCHOSOCIAL	
DESCRIBE MEMBERS OF SUPPORT SYSTEM OR IMMEDIATE HOUSEHOLD (AGE, HEALTH STATUS, ETC.) PATIENT'S RESPONSE TO CHANGE OR STRESS.	OBSERVED NON-VERBAL BEHAVIOR, INTERACTIONS WITH SIGNIFICANT OTHERS, ETC.

OCCUPATION AND/OR INTERESTS

DESCRIPTION OF HOME ENVIRONMENT

UTILIZATION OF COMMUNITY RESOURCES ☐ VNA ☐ PHN ☐ OTHER:	TYPE OF SERVICE PROVIDED

© ST. JOSEPH'S HOSPITAL - MILWAUKEE, WISCONSIN 1982

FORM 20523 1/82

SIGNATURE _____ RN

NURSING HISTORY & ASSESSMENT - PART B

FIGURE 1–3.   (cont.)

After reading Henderson's list of nursing activities, the nurse can readily adapt the list to a data collection format. For example, some of the following questions and observations relate to Henderson's activities:

Activity 1.   Breathe normally. The nurse counts the respirations, observes the depth of breathing, presence of retractions or nasal flaring, and uses a stethoscope to listen for lung sounds. The nurse may also ask the patient such questions as: Do you ever feel short of breath? What activity causes this? Do you have any allergies that make you congested or make it difficult to breathe? Do you ever experience nosebleeds? The nurse should also examine the nailbeds and extremities for color, warmth, and capillary refill; all these factors indicate the level of oxygenation.

Activity 2.   Eat and drink normally. The nurse may ask the patient to describe a normal day's diet, when the major meal of the day is taken, are there any foods that cause the patient problems, and to describe the resulting problems. The height, weight, and triceps skinfold may all be measured as a part of these data.

Following Henderson's framework, data related to each nursing activity should be collected in sequence.

Any format used for data collection is acceptable as long as it is thorough, comprehensive, and considers both the physiological and psychosocial aspects of the human being.

Data Collection Skills

At the time the patient is admitted to a health care facility, the nurse begins planning care for the patient. This is begun using the skills of data collection. Observation, interview, and examination are three methods the nurse uses to collect data. Although there are multiple sources the nurse may use to collect data, the patient is always the primary source. Even if the patient is unable to communicate verbally, the nurse can elicit valuable data using observation and examination skills. Additional data sources may be the patient's past medical record (chart), family members, and any other persons giving care to the patient. Professional journals, reference texts, and clinical nurse specialists are also important sources of data.

All nursing observations should result in objective data. *Objective data* are factual data that are observed by the nurse and could be noted by any other observer. The nurse describes the signs or behaviors ob-

Table 1-3

Objective Data	Judgments and Conclusions
Hair combed, makeup applied	Neatly groomed
Drags right leg when walking	Walks with slight limp
Tremors of both hands	Patient very afraid
250 cc dark amber urine	Large amount urine
Patient in bed, covers over head, facing wall; no verbal response to questions	Patient depressed
Administered own 8 A.M. insulin using sterile technique	Understands self administration of insulin
Ate cereal, juice, toast, coffee	Good appetite

served without drawing conclusions or making interpretations. See Table 1-3 for examples of objective data.

The column of judgments and conclusions demonstrates the interpretations of one individual nurse. Consider that "neatly groomed" may mean different things to different individuals, whereas "hair combed, makeup applied" is concise and descriptive.

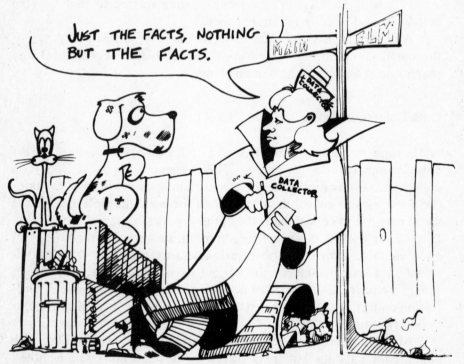

FIGURE 1-4.   The nurse records observations without drawing conclusions.

Contrasted with objective data are subjective data. *Subjective data* are information given verbally by the patient. Examples of this type of data are the following statements:

"I feel so nervous."
"My stomach is burning."
"I want to be alone now."

From the examples of subjective data listed above, each nurse could infer many different interpretations. For example, the nurse might guess that the patient was nervous, fearing a diagnosis of cancer. This interpretation is not justified on the basis of the patient's statement. The patient could be nervous for many different reasons. The task during the data collection phase is merely to observe, collect, and record data. Subjective data such as the examples in Table 1–4 are best recorded as direct quotes, thus providing the reader with the original information.

Table 1–4

Subjective Data	Judgments and Conclusions
"Get out of my room."	Hostile patient
"I know something is wrong with my baby."	Patient anxious
"This catheter is killing me."	Patient experiencing pain
"Where am I? How did I get here?"	Patient confused
"I'm afraid they will find cancer when they operate."	Patient worried about surgery

Observation.   Observation is a high-level nursing skill that requires a great deal of practice. Consider the party game where each participant is required to view a tray holding many items. After a brief period of time, the tray is removed and the participants are asked to list the items they can recall. Few people can successfully remember all the items. The skills of observation and recall are difficult. The inexperienced student will find it hard to perform nursing tasks and simultaneously continue the observation process. Yet it is this ability to perform constant, ongoing observations that is essential to assessment. For example, nursing students giving a first bedbath are concentrating so hard on the task that they are unable to make observations. As students gain skill in giving physical care, they can shift their attention to the total patient and begin to collect data through observation. They are now able to observe the skin condition, color, and temperature while bathing a patient. The quality, depth, and effort of respirations can be noted. The ability of the patient to move, as well as any pain with movement, is observed. While giving a back rub, the skilled student can view the skin over the lower back, which is often an area of breakdown. The condition of the mucous membrane is noted during oral hygiene. The ability of the patient to tolerate activity may also be observed as the nurse watches for signs of fatigue during and after the bath.

Interview.   The interview is a structured form of communication skill that the nurse uses to collect data. Both the ability to ask questions and the ability to listen are essential to the successful interview.

The nursing history is one type of interview. This is completed by the nurse at the time of admission. The focus on the nursing history is the patient's perception of current health status and unique response to it. In addition, the nurse reviews the client's past health history and coping methods that have been effectual or ineffectual. Data related to the patient's life-style may also help to identify health risk factors. The nursing history is not a duplicate of the medical history, which has the disease process as its main focus. The purpose of the nursing history is to enable the nurse to plan nursing care for the patient. The nurse clearly and directly conveys this purpose to the patient at the beginning of the interview. The nurse may something like, "Mr. Jones, I'd like to spend about half an hour with you talking about your health history. I have some questions to ask you. This information will help me to work with you to plan the nursing care you will receive during your hospitalization."

Prior to beginning the nursing history, the nurse helps to make the patient as comfortable as possible. It may be helpful to offer the patient the opportunity to go to the bathroom before beginning. Note that the nurse in the example above also gave the patient some indication of the amount of time the interview would take. This is helpful to the patient who may be expecting visitors or perhaps planning telephone calls. The nurse may also offer the patient a beverage if medically permitted. This may help to put the patient at ease and contribute to openness and recall in the interview process. It is also helpful if the nurse sits during the interview at a level where eye contact between the nurse and the patient can be easily maintained. This reduces the superior (nurse standing)-

inferior (patient in bed) feeling of the nurse-patient relationship and shows that the nurse has time to listen.

Most hospitals have a nursing history form that the nurse uses to guide the interview. This form is, however, only a starting point, and the nurse uses professional judgment to clarify areas of confusion or to elicit additional relevant data. The nurse will probably find it helpful to take brief notes during the interview process. Some explanation is always given to the patient. The nurse may say, "Mr. Jones, I'd like to take a few notes as we talk to be sure that I am accurate in recording this information." At the end of the interview it is helpful if the nurse summarizes the notes for the patient. This contributes to the development of trust in the nurse-patient relationship and gives the patient the opportunity to add or correct data.

Frequently, beginning nursing students are uncomfortable eliciting a nursing history. Students often state that they feel they are prying into personal matters. Students may be assured that the patient has the right to refuse to discuss any topic and that this right must be respected. When patients do reveal personal data, nurses and students are responsible for assuring that the shared information remains confidential. Such data will remain within the context of the relationship and will be shared only with those who need the information in order to provide care.

The formal nursing interview is not intended to be a treatment in and of itself, but is rather an organized format for data collection. Frequently, however, the patient has a need to express feelings, and the nursing interview provides the opportunity and the uninterrupted attention of the nurse. This is often therapeutic for the patient.

The informal aspect of the nursing interview is the conversation between the nurse and patient during the course of giving nursing care. The close relationship developed while the nurse is giving physical care frequently enables the patient to express feelings and problems. The nurse who can skillfully give physical care is then free to simultaneously focus attention on what the patient is saying.

The planned deliberate communication the nurse uses to help identify and meet the health care needs of the patient is called therapeutic communication. Like other nursing skills, therapeutic communication requires practice in order to be effective. It may be difficult for beginning nursing students to give physical care while simultaneously engaging in therapeutic communication. Often, for example, the nurse uses the time spent giving a bedbath as an opportunity for therapeutic communication. This is often an unhurried, private time for conversation between the nurse and patient. With practice, the nurse is able to focus on what the patient is expressing. During this communication the nurse continues to make observations.

At other times, the nurse will plan a period of time for the sole purpose of engaging in therapeutic communication. This, too, may be difficult for the beginning student, who may feel uncomfortable approaching patients without a technical skill (such as taking a blood pressure) to "do for" the patient. Often, however, therapeutic communication may be the only skill the nurse can offer the patient. This might be the case when a patient has just been told a life-threatening diagnosis.

Examination. The final activity of data collection is examination. Before beginning the physical process of examination, the nurse establishes a relationship with the patient. The nurse also precedes the examination by an introduction. The nurse then provides an explanation of the examination and requests the patient's permission to proceed. Provision for the patient's privacy (close both doors and curtains, please!) must be made.

The nurse is then ready to begin an examination of the patient. The nurse may choose to conduct a total body assessment or to focus on a specific area. For example, if a patient complains of generalized pain, the nurse may conduct a very thorough examination. In contrast, if a child in the emergency room fell from a bicycle and shows the nurse a large bleeding laceration on the elbow, this might be the initial focus of the examination. It is important though that the nurse conduct a thorough examination as soon as possible since internal injuries not so readily apparent may also be present.

In obtaining this examination data, the nurse uses a systematic approach in order to avoid omissions. The nurse may follow a cephalocaudal approach (meaning head to toe), which begins with an assessment of the hair, skull, eyes, ears, nose, mouth, and facial skin and moves in a downward direction. Another nurse may select a body systems approach, which may begin with a consideration of the respiratory system, moving to the digestive system, to the cardiovascular system, and so forth. Any methodical, thorough approach is acceptable as long as it meets the need to gather relevant data that helps to identify health problems requiring nursing intervention.

During physical examination the nurse uses several skills to collect data. *Visualization* is inspection of the client's body. This is coupled with the use of additional senses of the nurse such as hearing and smell. This is often the most appropriate starting place for a physical examination since the nurse will not cause the patient any discomfort, and the gentle touch of the nurse may enhance the relationship before the nurse continues with parts of the examination that may be more threatening to the client. The nurse also uses the skill of *auscultation*, which includes listening with a stethoscope to heart, lung, and bowel sounds. Next the nurse may *palpate* or feel the body. This may give the nurse information about organ position, body temperature, abnormal growths, abdominal rigidity, or the location of pain. Some nurses may be skilled in the use of *percussion*, the tapping of a body surface with a small rubber-tipped mallet or with the fingers. This is done in order to elicit responses, usually in the form of sound or movement, that give information about the underlying body part. For example, it is common practice to percuss a distended abdomen for a drumlike sound indicating retained flatus (gas) in the bowel following abdominal surgical procedures.

While it is necessary to establish a relationship with the patient prior to examination, the examination itself can also be a tool for showing concern and enhancing a relationship. The nurse who stops to palpate the abdomen and listen to bowel sounds when the patient complains of pain, shows concern for the patient and establishes credibility. The observations the nurse makes during an examination are recorded as objective data: 3-inch scar, left lower quadrant; temperature 98⁶F; BP 110/70; lungs sound normal and clear.

During the assessment phase the nurse has the potential to collect volumes of data about a client. Throughout the process it is important to consider the significance of the data to the task at hand, which is identifying problems and planning nursing intervention. As the student practices data collection, skill is gained in eliciting and recording relevant data.

DATA ANALYSIS

"So now that I've got all this data, what do I do with it?"
"Make sense out of it!"

The nurse has completed the initial systematic data collection and is now ready to begin the activity of analysis.

Analysis = Data Review + Data Interpretation

Data Review

The nurse now begins to consider all the data that were gathered during the assessment phase of the nursing process. The data must first be organized into some useful format. If the form used to collect the data was based on a particular nursing framework, the data may already be organized in a useful format. Using Maslow's basic needs as a format for data collection, the nurse may review the data and notice, for example, that no data on rest and sleep patterns are included. This would point out the need to go back and gather additional data. In this example the data review has helped the nurse to identify an error of omission.

The nurse also looks for inconsistencies in the data. It may become apparent to the nurse that the sequence of events in the health history is in contradiction and needs to be resolved. Another example might be that the nurse is unclear from reading the data what methods the patient has used for pain relief and with what result. There may also be an inconsistency between two data sources. For example, the patient may report having only an occasional "social drink" while the spouse gives data about "drinking 6 to 12 cans of beer daily." At this point no judgment is made about the existence of a problem, but the inconsistency is noted.

The data are evaluated for comprehensiveness, for a holistic approach. The nurse questions whether the assessment has considered all areas that may be relevant to the patient. This considers such things as cultural data, data related to growth and development, and psychosocial factors as well as the more obvious physical areas. These factors taken together comprise holistic health, that is, the concept that the mind and the body are inseparable and that one cannot be treated without the other.

In summary, the nurse reviews the data for

—organization
—inconsistencies
—comprehensiveness.

Data Interpretation

Up to this point the nurse has reviewed the data without making any judgments or conclusions. Now the nurse studies the data and makes judgments, conclusions, and decisions about the meaning of the data.

The nurse considers the data and decides whether one piece of information (or sign, symptom, measurement) is sufficient to warrant a focus for nursing intervention or whether the data require further study and relating to additional data. A slightly elevated blood pressure unaccompanied by other data may not be significant, whereas the auscultation of abnormal lung sounds requires nursing intervention even without additional data.

The following decisions are reached based on the data:

1. Determine whether measurement data are within the normal range for the client. For example, if the nurse has taken the blood pressure of the patient, the nurse can now relate this to other data such as age, weight, and sex and make a decision as to the status of the client.

2. Evaluate the physical assessment data for positive, negative, normal, or abnormal signs or findings. If the nurse has completed auscultation of the patient's lungs, the nurse includes a description of whether the findings were normal and, if not, which particular abnormality was heard. The statement that a particular aspect of the assessment was negative is valuable in that it notes that a judgment has been made and a potential problem area ruled out.

3. Determine whether specific behavior patterns contribute to the health and well-being of the client. The nurse may evaluate that dietary and exercise patterns of the client foster cardiovascular health as in the case of a patient who reports that she has never smoked, exercises three times per week, and has decreased intake of red meat to twice a week. The nurse also considers the opposite possibility; determine what factors the client possesses that negatively affect health status.

4. Determine what strengths or resources the client possesses that affect health status. For example, the nurse may make the judgment that the client whose assessment data indicate a current YMCA membership has a potential resource affecting health status. Another patient who has suffered a mild heart attack may indicate, "That was a warning. Now I'm ready to do whatever I have to to get healthy and stay healthy." The nurse may interpret these data as a willingness to receive health teaching and a motivation to follow through.

After a thorough review of the data has been completed, the nurse continues by examining the data to determine whether relationships exist between the pieces of data. For example, if the data reveal that the patient has high blood pressure, is overweight by 25%, and has no understanding of caloric requirements and content, the nurse begins to see a relationship between factors that all contribute to health problems. The nurse then "filters" the related data through the body of nursing knowledge and uses this to identify problem areas. At this time the nurse does not attempt to make a specific statement of the problem. The nurse does list a focus of attention, a broad area that requires further refinement or clarification. This might be compared to adjusting the focus on a movie projector for greater clarity.

For example, the nurse may read data that includes such things as a history of being overweight since childhood, "My Mother used to bake me a double whipped-cream cake if I got a good report card," "I've tried every diet in the book," "I don't really like being so fat but aren't fat people supposed to be jolly?" "My children are plump, but it's just baby fat and they'll grow out of it," patient is aged 29 years, 5 feet, 2 inches, weighs 189 pounds. The nurse uses a knowledge of normal nutrition, behavioral psychology, and growth and development in considering these data. This data cluster indicates a focus for nursing intervention in the area of nutrition.

The nurse may review the listing of accepted nursing diagnoses in Table 1-5 and select "alteration in nutrition" as a focus. Later the nurse will refine this to be more specific.

Another patient assessment may include the following data: pain in the lower back, unable to perform job (cashier in grocery store) because it causes pain, cannot do any housework without causing aggravation of pain, "My Mother had a bad back and she was an invalid at age 45." Here the nurse also applies the knowledge of related sciences to recognize that the data indicate an area for nursing intervention. Again, consulting Table 1-5 the nurse might state the focus as "alteration in comfort," and "disturbance in self-esteem." Again, this will be refined and clarified later in the statement of the nursing diagnosis.

Table 1-5   Approved Nursing Diagnoses

Activity intolerance
Activity intolerance, potential
Airway clearance, ineffective
Anxiety
Bowel elimination, alteration in: constipation
Bowel elimination, alteration in: diarrhea
Bowel elimination, alteration in: incontinence
Breathing pattern, ineffective
Cardiac output, alteration in: decreased
Comfort, alteration in: pain
Communication, impaired: verbal
Coping, family: potential for growth

Table 1-5 Approved Nursing Diagnoses (cont.)

Coping, ineffective family: compromised
Coping, ineffective family: disabling
Coping, ineffective individual
Diversional activity, deficit
Family process, alteration in
Fear
Fluid volume, alteration in: excess
Fluid volume deficit, actual
Fluid volume deficit, potential
Gas exchange, impaired
Grieving, anticipatory
Grieving, dysfunctional
Health maintenance, alteration in
Home maintenance mangement, impaired
Injury, potential for (poisoning, potential for; suffocation, potential for; trauma, potential for)
Knowledge deficit (specify)
Mobility, impaired physical
Noncompliance (specify)
Nutrition, alteration in: less than body requirements
Nutrition, alteration in: more than body requirements
Nutrition, alteration in: potential for more than body requirements
Oral mucous membrane, alteration in
Parenting, alteration in: actual
Parenting, alteration in: potential
Powerlessness
Rape trauma syndrome
Self-care deficit: feeding, bathing/hygiene, dressing/grooming, toileting
Self-concept, disturbance in: body image, self-esteem, role performance, personal identity
Sensory-perceptual alteration: visual, auditory, kinesthetic, gustatory, tactile, olfactory
Sexual dysfunction
Skin integrity, impairment of: actual
Skin integrity, impairment of: potential
Sleep pattern disturbance
Social isolation
Spiritual distress (distress of the human spirit)
Thought processes, alteration in
Tissue perfusion, alteration in: cerebral, cardiopulmonary, renal, gastrointestinal, peripheral
Urinary elimination, alteration in patterns
Violence, potential for: self-directed or directed at others

From *Classification of Nursing Diagnoses*, Proceedings of the Fifth National Conference, edited by Mi Ja Kim, Gertrude K. McFarland, and Audrey M. McLane. Mosby, St. Louis, 1984.

It may be helpful for the student to turn to the *Nursing Diagnosis Pocketbook* for further aids in identifying the focus area.

NURSING DIAGNOSIS

The final step in the assessment process is the formulation of nursing diagnoses. In a five-step nursing process format, interpretation of data and determination of nursing diagnoses are part of the analysis step, as are priority setting and selection of patient care goals. These activities are discussed in Chapter 2 of this text as part of the planning step.

NURSING DIAGNOSIS:

A statement of a present or potential patient problem that requires nursing intervention in order to be resolved, or lessened, or adapted to.

The nurse begins the process of writing nursing diagnoses by reviewing the focus area identified in the previous step. Does the focus area represent a problem? By definition, a nursing diagnosis must be a problem. If it is not a problem, no nursing diagnosis need be made. Consider the bowel function status of a patient restricted to bedrest. If the patient has a soft, formed stool without exertion every 2 to 3 days, elimination is not a problem and no nursing diagnosis need be made. However, the nurse must also consider who defines a problem. If the patient considers it abnormal not to have a daily bowel movement and continues to express anxiety related to this, a problem does exist as defined by the patient. The nurse may understand that physiologically no problem exists, but that the patient could benefit from teaching regarding normal body function. Nursing care may then focus on teaching as an intervention tool to reduce anxiety.

Types of Nursing Diagnoses

As defined here, the problem expressed in the nursing diagnosis may be either present or potential. A *present nursing diagnosis* refers to a situation existing in the here and now. A patient on a general diet with a good appetite has not had a bowel movement for 4 days, complains of low abdominal pain, and is unable to pass stool. This patient is constipated and requires assistance. This is a current problem for the patient.

A *potential nursing diagnosis* refers to a problem which may develop in the future. By identifying the potential problem, the nurse may be able to prevent the problem or lessen its consequences. If a patient is on absolute bedrest while in a full leg cast, the patient is at risk for developing bedsores (decubitus ulcers) related to inactivity and decreased circulation. Understanding the physiological effects of bedrest, the nurse may take action to prevent bed sores. In this case, the problem is a potential one that requires preventive nursing intervention. The potential nursing diagnosis is made based on the nurse's past experience in similar situations and on an understanding of pathophysiology. The problem would predictably occur without nursing intervention.

In still other situations, the nurse may wish to formulate a *tentative*, or possible *nursing diagnosis*. This type of nursing diagnosis may be made when the nurse has insufficient data from an individual patient to support a firm nursing diagnosis. This may be compared to the physician who lists several "rule out" medical diagnoses in a patient's admission assessment. By considering such a tentative nursing diagnosis, the nurse assures continued collection of relevant data. With an increased database, the nurse may be able to firmly establish the tentative nursing diagnosis as valid or to eliminate the tentative nursing diagnosis as invalid for this particular patient. For example:

> An adolescent has arrived in the emergency room to receive stitches for a scalp laceration. Treatment requires that a large portion of her head be shaved. The nurse considers a tentative nursing diagnosis of disturbance in self-esteem related to loss of hair. The nurse bases this diagnosis on her knowledge of growth and development, since most adolescents are very concerned about their physical appearance. Note, however, that this diagnosis is not supported by data from this individual patient. This diagnosis is based on inference at this point and thus is tentative. The nurse seeks to gather more data as she asks the patient, "A lot of girls might be very upset about having their hair cut. How do you feel about this?" The patient replies, "No problem, I wear lots of wigs." The nurse may then eliminate that tentative diagnosis.

The nurse also considers a second criterion when beginning to write nursing diagnoses: does the problem require nursing intervention in order to be resolved, lessened, or adapted to? The nurse may identify problems that are clearly within the realm of another health professional. In such a case the nurse communicates the data to that professional but rules out a nursing diagnosis.

Writing Nursing Diagnoses

The following formula will result in a clear, concise statement of a nursing diagnosis.

Nursing Diagnosis = Patient Problem + Cause If Known

Nothing, repeat, nothing else, belongs in the nursing diagnosis. Keep it clean! When beginning it may be helpful to state a nursing diagnosis and then identify the data on which the nursing diagnosis is based. This helps to assure that a nursing diagnosis is accurate and is based on facts. A nursing diagnosis is not an inference. If you are unable to identify the data on which a nursing diagnosis is based, there are two alternatives. You may go back and collect more data, or you may write a tentative nursing diagnosis to assure the continuance of data collection. Both alternatives stress the necessity of supporting the nursing diagnosis by using data. The following suggestions may also guide you in formulating nursing diagnoses:

1. Keep nursing diagnoses brief.
2. Keep nursing diagnoses specific.
3. Each nursing diagnosis relates to one patient problem.
4. Each nursing diagnosis must be based on patient data.

The nurse is now ready to begin writing nursing diagnoses. It may be helpful at this time to refer to the appendix of this text. After identifying the focus of nursing intervention, the nurse can locate an approved nursing diagnosis, its definition, defining characteristics, and possible etiologies (cause). Nursing diagnoses need not be limited to those included in Appendix B, the *Nursing Diagnosis Pocketbook*.

The following examples combine these elements to form nursing diagnoses.

Problem	+	*Cause if Known*	=	*Nursing Diagnosis*
1. Pain		Associated with surgical incision		Alteration in comfort: pain related to incision
2. Unable to bathe self		Related to decreased activity tolerance		Self-care deficit: bathing, level 2, secondary to decreased activity tolerance
3. Difficulty breathing		Related pulmonary congestion		Ineffective breathing pulmonary congestion
4. Boredom		Related to isolation precautions		Diversional activity deficit related to isolation precautions
5. Fear		Related to uncertain diagnosis		Fear related to uncertain diagnosis
6. Unable to sleep		Related to fear of surgery		Sleep pattern disturbance related to fear of surgery

A nursing diagnosis is not synonymous with a medical diagnosis. The following comparison may help to clarify what constitutes a nursing diagnosis. Note that the cause of a problem is usually not a medical diagnosis. The cause portion of a nursing diagnosis is intended to give direction to nursing intervention. A medical diagnosis as a cause is of limited value in directing nursing care.

A Nursing Diagnosis	
Is	*Is Not*
A statement of a patient problem	A medical diagnosis
Actual or potential	A nursing action
Within the scope of nursing intervention	A physician's order
Suggestive of nursing intervention	A therapeutic treatment

Frequently a medical diagnosis may suggest nursing diagnoses.

Medical Diagnosis	Nursing Diagnosis
Peptic ulcer	Alteration in comfort: pain related to peptic ulcer
Myocardial infarction	Fear related to possible recurrence of myocardial infarction
Cerebral vascular accident	Self-care deficit: dressing/grooming, level 1, related to cerebral vascular accident
Chronic ulcerative colitis	Alteration in bowel elimination, diarrhea related to CUC
Cancer of the breast	Body image disturbance related to mastectomy.
Senile bilateral cataract	Potential for injury related to poor vision.

Table 1–5 lists the nursing diagnoses that are currently accepted by the North American Nursing Diagnosis Association. These problem statements are intended to provide an initial standardized listing of nursing diagnoses. The listing is by no means complete but represents a beginning standardization of nursing diagnoses. It is hoped that such a listing will expand the body of nursing knowledge, provide a basis for nursing research into nursing diagnosis, and provide a means of communicating nursing diagnoses among nurses. Although the list is very helpful, beginning students are cautioned not to get bogged down by difficulties with "saying it right." When beginning, state the problem in your own words in a way that communicates clearly and concisely. Do not hesitate to add your problem statements to the listing.

Practice Exercise

Pick out the correctly written nursing diagnoses. Identify what is wrong with the incorrectly written nursing diagnoses. The answers are on the following pages.

1. Alteration in nutrition: less than body requirements related to nausea following chemotherapy.
2. Range of motion (ROM) exercises associated with stroke.
3. Cancer of the breast related to primary site.
4. Refusing wound irrigation related to pain of procedure.

5. Body image disturbance related to amputation of right foot.
6. Prone to altered sexual identity and sexual behavior in relating to husband and friends secondary to mastectomy.
7. Intermittent positive pressure breathing (IPPB) exercises q.i.d. to increase lung expansion.
8. Alteration in comfort: pain and fear related to surgical procedure.
9. Severe itching related to fungal infection.
10. Activity intolerance related to difficulty ambulating.
11. Impaired physical mobility associated with right side paralysis.
12. Ineffective breathing pattern, etiology unknown.
13. Disorientation to time and place related to confused state.
14. Impaired verbal communication related to native Spanish language.
15. Anxiety related to nervous tension.
16. Ambulate progressively q.i.d. with tripod cane.
17. Potential for infection related to second-degree burns.
18. Patient is upset and worried about health problems.
19. Impaired skin integrity secondary to prolonged bedrest.
20. Thrombophlebitis related to prolonged bedrest.

Answers to Exercise on Nursing Diagnosis

Evaluation	*Rationale*
1. Correct	Problem = less than body requirements for nutrition Cause = nausea following chemotherapy
2. Incorrect	ROM exercises are a nursing action.
3. Incorrect	This is a medical diagnosis.
4. Incorrect	This is a nursing problem, not a patient problem.
5. Correct	Problem = body image disturbance Cause = amputation of right foot
6. Incorrect	Vague and nonspecific Multiple problems Too long
7. Incorrect	This is a medical treatment.
8. Incorrect	Two separate problems

   9. Correct   Problem = severe itching
                    Cause   = fungal infection

  10. Incorrect   Problem and cause are the same.

  11. Incorrect   Problem and cause are the same.

  12. Correct   Problem = ineffective breathing
                    Cause   = unknown

  13. Incorrect   Problem and cause are the same.

  14. Correct   Problem = impaired verbal communication
                    Cause   = native Spanish language

  15. Incorrect   Problem and cause are the same.

  16. Incorrect   This is a physician's order.

  17. Correct   Problem = potential for infection
                    Cause   = second-degree burns

  18. Incorrect   Vague and nonspecific

  19. Correct   Problem = impaired skin integrity
                    Cause   = prolonged bedrest

  20. Incorrect   Thrombophlebitis is a medical diagnosis.

The case study method will be used through this book to illustrate
the steps of the nursing process. The same case study of Mrs. Witten
will be found in each chapter to illustrate the various steps in the nursing process. The following pages illustrate the nursing assessment that
was done for Mrs. Witten and the nursing diagnoses derived from the
data. The final chapter will include the nursing care plan as it might appear in a hospital Kardex or similar list of patient care plans.

MRS. WITTEN: NURSING DIAGNOSES

1. Alteration in comfort: acute pain related to probable gallbladder disease.

2. Fear related to uncertain outcome and hospitalization.

3. Knowledge deficit: insufficient knowledge related to surgical
   treatment.

4. Health management deficit: inability to perform breast self-
   examination related to lack of knowledge.

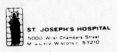

ST JOSEPH'S HOSPITAL
5000 West Chambers Street
Milwaukee Wisconsin 53210

NURSING HISTORY & ASSESSMENT

Mrs. Laura Witten
365-8976-2635
Dr. Ronal/Keller
Room 621

PART A

(MEDICAL · SURGICAL)

DATE OF HISTORY	TIME OF HISTORY	INFORMANT(S)
6/3-86	8 PM (2000 hours)	MRS. LAURA WITTEN (& hsb Bob)

ADMITTING MEDICAL DIAGNOSIS
R/O Cholecystitis / Cholelithiasis

ARRIVED ON UNIT: ☐ AMBULATORY ☑ WHEELCHAIR ☐ CART ☐ AMBULANCE

REASONS FOR HOSPITALIZATION
Severe pain in right upper quadrant. "It has never been this bad before".

HOW HAS THE PATIENT BEEN MANAGING THE ABOVE PROBLEMS AT HOME?
Usually goes away after a couple hours

OTHER ILLNESSES OR CONDITIONS (HYPERTENSION, ARTHRITIS, DIABETES, PAST SURGERIES, ETC.)
none

ALLERGIES (FOOD, MEDICATION, TAPE, DYE, ETC.)
none known

ALCOHOL USAGE	LAST PHYSICAL EXAM	TYPE OF REACTION
One or two glasses wine/day	6 mo. ago	NA

MEDICATION AND DOSAGE PRESCRIBED AND NON-PRESCRIBED	USUAL TIMES TAKEN	TIME OF LAST DOSE	PATIENT'S UNDERSTANDING OF PURPOSE
none			

SUBJECTIVE DATA	OBJECTIVE DATA

COGNITION/SENSATION/COMMUNICATION

LIMITATIONS OR RESTRICTIONS RELATED TO:
VISION: ☑ YES ☐ NO   HEARING: ☐ YES ☐ NO   OTHER: ☐ YES ☐ NO
DESCRIBE:
"Can't see a thing without them – not even the big E on the eye chart."
LAST EYE EXAM: 2 years ago

LEVEL OF ORIENTATION (ALERTNESS, ABILITY TO PROCESS INFORMATION, ETC.)
Oriented and able to respond to questions

GLASSES ☑
CONTACT LENSES ☑
ARTIFICIAL EYE
HEARING AID

APPEARANCE OF EYES, EARS, SPEECH IMPAIRMENTS, ETC.
Normal

VENTILATION

REPORT OF DYSPNEA/COUGH, ORTHOPNEA, ETC
no cough, no shortness of breath
HOW MUCH DOES PATIENT SMOKE? none

BREATH SOUNDS, SPUTUM, ETC.
Lungs clear
RESP RATE 28   DEPTH & QUALITY ↑ depth

ST. JOSEPH'S HOSPITAL, MILWAUKEE, WISCONSIN 1982

SIGNATURE _____ M. E. Murray _____ R.N.

NURSING HISTORY & ASSESSMENT · PART A

FORM 20441 REV. 5/84

FIGURE 1–5. Assessment form. Courtesy of St. Joseph's Hospital, Milwaukee, Wisconsin.

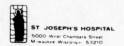

ST. JOSEPH'S HOSPITAL
5000 West Chambers Street
Milwaukee Wisconsin 53210

NURSING
HISTORY &
ASSESSMENT

(MEDICAL-SURGICAL)

Mrs. Laura Witten
365-8976-2635
Dr. Ronal/Keller
Room 621

PART B

SUBJECTIVE DATA	OBJECTIVE DATA
CIRCULATION — REPORT OF CHEST PAIN, NUMBNESS, TINGLING, ETC. "No chest pain, numbness, tingling"	PERIPHERAL PULSES, CAPILLARY REFILL, HOMAN'S SIGN, EDEMA, ETC. Brisk capillary refill, neg. Homan's TEMP 99⁸ ☒ O ☐ AX ☐ R PULSES ☐ AP ☐ R _____ QUALITY _____ BP 158/88 ☐ R ☒ L ☒ LYING ☐ SITTING ☐ STANDING
NUTRITION/ HYDRATION — REPORTS OF ANOREXIA, NAUSEA, USUAL MEAL PATTERN, ABILITY TO CHEW AND SWALLOW, RECENT CHANGE IN WEIGHT, ETC. c/o nausea now. "Put on 20 lbs over past 5 years" THERAPEUTIC DIET none LAST DENTAL EXAM 8 mo.	SKIN TURGOR, APPEARANCE OF TONGUE, CONDITION OF TEETH, ETC. Mucous membranes intact White teeth - several fillings noted HEIGHT 5'6" WEIGHT 145 DENTURES none
ELIMINATION — BOWEL HABITS, VOIDING PATTERN, HEMORRHOIDS, DESCRIPTION OF MENSTRUAL CYCLE, ETC. Daily BM - regular 29 day menstrual cycle REPORTED LBM this am LAST PAP SMEAR 6 mo. ago LAST PROCTOSCOPIC EXAM none	DIAPHORESIS, BOWEL SOUNDS, APPEARANCE OF URINE, FECES, VOMITUS, ETC. Clear, light amber urine. No emesis. Moderate diaphoresis.
MOBILITY — REPORTED INABILITY TO DO ADLS, DIFFICULTY WITH AMBULATION, ETC. Able to walk without assistance	ROM, GAIT, STRENGTH, ENDURANCE, ETC. Splints side c̄ hands when asked to move CANE _____ CRUTCHES _____ WALKER _____ PROSTHESIS _____
INTEGUMENTARY — REPORTED PRURITIS, ECZEMA, PSORIASIS, ETC. "My skin is very dry. I use LAST SELF-BREAST EXAM never learned" lots of moisture cream."	INSPECTION FOR RASHES, OPEN AREAS, AND ABNORMAL NAIL CONDITION, ETC. NOTE DISTRIBUTION AND QUALITY OF HAIR OR PRESENCE OF WIG Skin intact, good color. Hair clean, no dandruff, no rash.
COMFORT SLEEP - REST — REPORT OF PAIN, QUALITY, LOCATION, PRECIPITATING FACTORS, DURATION AND HOW PAIN IS RELIEVED Hurts here - I can't stand it - never been so bad." REPORTED SLEEP PATTERNS AND BEDTIME RITUALS 7-8 hours/night. Bed @ 11 PM	FACIAL GRIMACING, GUARDING OF AFFECTED AREA, ETC. (NOTE: THERE MAY BE NO OBSERVABLE SIGNS WITH CHRONIC PAIN.) Clenching hands, gritting teeth, restless. Points to RUQ to locate pain.
PSYCHOSOCIAL — DESCRIBE MEMBERS OF SUPPORT SYSTEM OR IMMEDIATE HOUSEHOLD (AGE, HEALTH STATUS, ETC.) PATIENT'S RESPONSE TO CHANGE OR STRESS. "I've never been in a hospital before. I'm really scared. I've never even had my tonsils out".	OBSERVED NON-VERBAL BEHAVIOR, INTERACTIONS WITH SIGNIFICANT OTHERS, ETC. Slightly weepy & hands trembling. Husband present.

OCCUPATION AND/OR INTERESTS Buyer for dept. store. Likes to read, walk dog, sing in church choir.

DESCRIPTION OF HOME ENVIRONMENT Lives in single family home in suburb. "My sons (ages 15,13) really depend on me for transportation everywhere."

UTILIZATION OF COMMUNITY RESOURCES ☐ VNA ☐ PHN ☐ OTHER: none   TYPE OF SERVICE PROVIDED none

ⓒ ST. JOSEPH'S HOSPITAL - MILWAUKEE, WISCONSIN 1982

FORM 20523 1/82

SIGNATURE _____ M. E. Murray _____ RN

NURSING HISTORY & ASSESSMENT - PART B

FIGURE 1–5. (cont.)

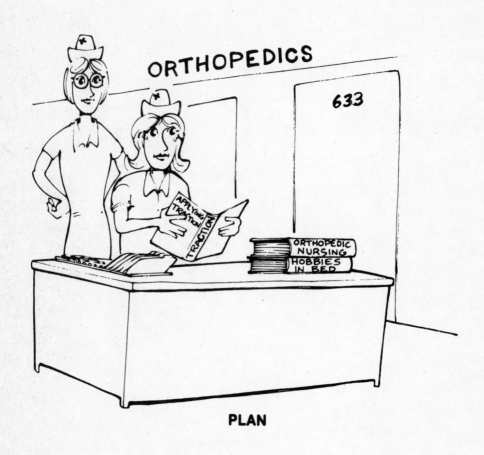

PLAN

CHAPTER 2

Planning

Now that you have collected data about your patient, analyzed that data, and formulated some nursing diagnoses, you are ready to begin the planning phase of the nursing process. In the planning phase, the nurse develops a plan to assist the patient to an optimum or improved level of functioning in the problem areas identified in the nursing diagnoses. The nurse analyzes the strengths and weaknesses of the patient, the patient's family, the nursing personnel, the health care facility, and the available resources (including other health professionals).

A plan is developed to make nursing care both individualized for the patient and realistic for the health care or home care setting. The skills of problem solving and decision making are applied to a particular patient's identified problems. The resulting plan of nursing care is designed to help patients and their families:

—maintain their current level of health and functioning if they are identified at risk for developing problems
—reach an improved level of health and functioning
—adjust to a reduced level of health when cure is not possible
—adjust as well as possible to a terminal illness.

There are three steps in the planning phase: setting priorities among the nursing diagnoses when a patient has several problems, establishing goals with a patient, and planning specific nursing interventions to help a patient achieve the goals.

Planning = Setting Priorities + Establishing Goals + Planning Nursing Interventions

---

SETTING PRIORITIES

During the process of priority setting, the nurse and the patient, whenever possible, determine which problems identified during the assessment phase are in need of immediate attention and which problems might be dealt with at a later time. Consider assigning identified patient problems a high, middle, or low priority. The higher-priority problems deserve the most immediate nursing attention for a plan and treatment. Setting priorities serves the purpose of ordering the delivery of nursing care so that more important problems are considered before lesser ones. Priority setting does not mean that one problem must be totally resolved before another problem is considered. Problems can frequently be approached simultaneously.

Guidelines for Setting Priorities

1. Maslow's hierarchy of basic needs can guide your selection of high-priority problems. Survival needs that are significantly unmet pose the greatest threat to life and functioning and thus deserve a high priority rating. Using Maslow's theory to guide the delivery of nursing care, the nurse would:

    > Relieve a patient's pain (physiological need) before encouraging morning hygiene (self-esteem). Encourage a new mother to talk about her experience in labor (self-esteem need) before expecting her to take on the new role of mothering with great involvement (self-actualization need). Stabilize bleeding and ensure adequate oxygenation in an emergency room accident victim before assessing elimination status (both of these are basic physiological needs, but oxygenation is usually the highest priority need; bleeding is considered a threat to tissue oxygen needs).

    Consider how difficult it is for you to read and absorb the material in this book (self-actualization need) if you have had too little sleep (physiological need). Basic survival needs will usually take priority over higher-level needs if the survival needs are not being satisfied. This is the case when a patient is in obvious physical distress owing to the unmet need. If the survival needs are being partially met and actual physical distress is minimal, a higher-level need may take priority or at least have the same priority as a lower-level need. For example, an auto accident victim can be in considerable distress with multiple physical needs unmet, yet the priority need may be to ascertain the whereabouts and injuries of the other family members in the car when it crashed. This unmet higher-level need can have a negative effect on satisfaction of this patient's physical needs if it is not given appropriate attention.

2. Focus on the problems the patient feels are most important if this priority does not interfere with medical treatment. A patient's need for undisturbed rest cannot take precedence over a medical treatment that requires the observation of blood pressure and pulse every hour following a car accident. If there are no contraindications, offer patients the opportunity to set their own priorities. This serves two purposes. First, this approach involves patients in planning their own care. Perhaps the nurse has overlooked a major problem that is consuming the patient's time and energy or has assigned the problem a low priority. Unless this problem is considered first, the nurse may be able to achieve only limited success in other areas because the patient is still worrying about the overlooked prob-

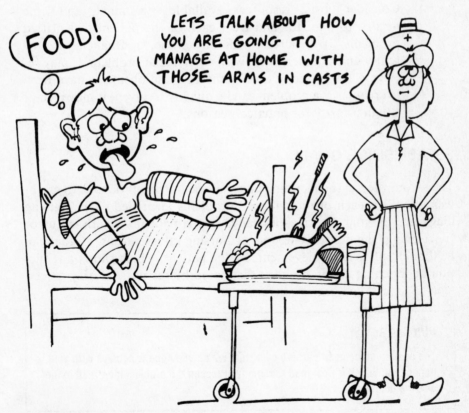

FIGURE 2–1. Priority setting.

lem. Second, cooperation between the nurse and the patient is enhanced when priority setting is done together.

3. Consider the effect of potential problems when setting priorities. For example:

> A new mother may ask to be left alone with her husband and newborn to get acquainted. The potential problem of a postpartum hemorrhage would require continuous observation after delivery, since this is potentially life threatening. Thus the patient's request to be left alone cannot be safely met.
>
> A bedridden patient may be started on a routine of frequent turning and positioning to prevent bed sores and contractures, even though the patient may not see this as important. Prevention of the potential complications of prolonged bedrest is a high priority.

Prevention of a potential problem, rather than treatment of the problem when it develops, is a goal deserving continuous assessment and intervention.

4. Consider costs, resources available, personnel, and time needed to plan for and treat each of the patient's identified problems. If resources, personnel, time, or financing is currently unavailable to deal with a particular problem, it may receive a low priority until some of these obstacles have been overcome. If a problem can be quickly resolved, it may receive a high priority for practical reasons.

ESTABLISHING GOALS

The second step in the planning phase of the nursing process is to establish a goal for each of the patient's problems identified in the nursing diagnoses. A goal describes a change in the patient's health status or functioning: the desired outcome of nursing interventions. A goal can be thought of as an achievement, by the patient, which shows a reduction or lessening of the problem diagnosed by the nurse during assessment.

NURSING GOAL:

The desired outcome of nursing care; that which you hope to achieve with your patient and which is designed to remedy or lessen the problem identified in the nursing diagnosis.

Why Do I Need A Goal Statement?

You need a goal as part of your plan of care because it gives guidance to the type of nursing interventions you will choose. A goal is a constant reminder of why you are doing what you are doing with each patient. Goals will give you a sense of timing as you gauge your patient's hourly, daily, weekly, monthly, yearly, and lifelong efforts to maintain and improve health and functioning. Goals give you a sense of where this particular patient started from and where the individual and the nurse hope to end up. The goals you write will be the criteria you use to evaluate the success of your nursing interventions. A goal helps to motivate both the nurse and the patient to continue their efforts. When goals are achieved, it provides the patient, the patient's family, and the nurse and other caregivers with the reward of success, and success promotes further efforts to achieve other goals.

The goal area in a sporting event is always clearly identified. It would be very difficult to give a field goal kicker in football credit for a field goal without a goalpost. The same is true in nursing. Without a clear, concise goal statement, the nurse and the patient do not know if and when the desired end has been achieved. A goal statement in nursing should be as clearly defined as the end zone in football.

The Standards of Nursing Practice identified by the American Nurses' Association state, "The plan of nursing care includes goals derived from the nursing diagnoses." The professional nurse is expected to demonstrate the ability to develop and communicate goals as part of each patient's care. The Joint Commission of American Hospitals, which is the national organization for accrediting hospitals, identifies, as one of their standards for approving a hospital, "Individualized, goal-directed nursing care shall be provided through the use of the nursing process."

Time Frameworks for Goal Achievement—Long- and Short-Term Goals

All goals include a time at which point the patient is to be evaluated for goal achievement. Goals can be classified as short- and long-term goals based on the length of time the patient is given to accomplish the behavior identified in the goal. The nurse may feel that some goals are so critical to patient survival that goal achievement is hoped for in terms of hours or less. Other goals dealing with optimum recovery from health problems may span years.

Short-Term Goals. Short-term goals identify outcomes in patients' status or behavior that can be achieved fairly quickly, in a matter of hours or days. Short-term goals are especially appropriate to acute-care settings, such as intensive care units, emergency rooms, recovery rooms, to name a few. Patients in these settings are unstable, and their physical status is often changing rapidly. The long-term prognosis for these patients is uncertain, and health care is focused on the present.

If a problem is diagnosed that tends to worsen with the passage of time, short-term goals are more appropriate than long-term goals. The nurse wants to see a change in patient behavior soon; the problem cannot be allowed to continue until physical or psychological damage occurs. For example, the patient who is unable to void following surgery cannot be left for 24 hours with a filling bladder. Extreme discomfort and possible rupture of the bladder would be the consequence. A short-term goal is identified for a patient following surgery, such as "reestablishment of urinary elimination within 6 to 8 hours after surgery." If the patient is unable to achieve this goal, a catheter is often inserted to empty the bladder and prevent damage.

Some examples of short-term goals are the following:

Newborn's respirations below 70 breaths/minute within 1 hour.
Return of bowel sounds within 12 hours postop.
Passing flatus within 24 hours postop.
Temperature to be below 102°F within 1 hour.
Fetal heart rate to remain normal during labor and delivery.
For the reader of this book: Completion of Chapter 2 within the
    next hour.

When you start to write goals, start with short-term goals. As a beginning nursing student, you are not with the same patient for long periods of time. You may care for the patient for only 1 or 2 days. If you write a short-term goal involving the length of time you plan to be with the patient, you will be able to give the needed nursing care and evaluate the results yourself. By evaluating whether your goal was met before you leave the patient, you will gain skill in writing realistic goals and in giving nursing care to meet those goals.

Short-term goals are often developed to help the nurse and the patient gauge progress toward long-term goals. By achieving short-term goals, the patient is gradually advanced to the improved level of functioning identified in the long-term goal. Achievement of short-term goals provides repeated satisfaction for both the nurse and the patient, serving as evidence of progress and guidance for the future. For example, the nurse and the patient have identified a long-term goal, "weight loss of 80 pounds in 1 year." Progressive short-term goals are identified to help the nurse and the patient measure progress toward long-term goal achievement. For example,

Weight of 210 pounds by February 7
Weight of 208 pounds by February 14
Weight of 206 pounds by February 21

A series of shorter-term goals that a person can realistically accomplish in a stated time period is much more rewarding than striving for one long-term goal. The repeated reinforcement a person receives from meeting shorter-term goals can keep an individual motivated to achieve a long-term goal.

Some other examples of short-term goals leading to a long-term goal are the following:

1. "I will finish reading this book before final exams" might be a long-term goal for a student in nursing. This student might accomplish the long-term goal by progressive short-term goals of reading one chapter each week.
2. "Patient will demonstrate full use of broken arm within 6 months." This patient might accomplish the long-term goal by progressively increasing the amount and range of muscle/joint exercises.
3. "Performance of self-care activities within 3 months of cerebral vascular accident (stroke)." Progressive short-term goals might focus on accomplishment of one self-care activity a week until the patient was able to perform many activities independently.
   Week of 10/10: Feeds self by end of week.
   Week of 10/17: Brushing teeth by end of week.
   Week of 10/24: Performs personal hygiene by end of week.
   Week of 10/31: Meets own mobility needs by end of week.

Long-Term Goals. Long-term goals give direction for nursing care over time. Long-term goals try to identify the maximum level of functioning possible for a patient with a particular diagnosed problem. Consider the prognosis of the patient's health problems, resources available, strengths and weakness of the patient and family, and nursing care abilities of personnel who will be working with the patient. If the patient has an alteration in some function, the long-term goal is to restore a normal pattern of functioning, if possible. If that is not possible, the goal deals with establishing a maximum level of functioning for the alteration and assisting the patient to adjust to this altered level of functioning. Some examples of long-term goals are the following:

> Reestablishment of normal bowel elimination patterns in 2 months.
> Maintenance of skin integrity during period of immobility.
> Breastfeeding 10 to 15 minutes/breast, every 2 to 5 hours, within 1 week of delivery.
> Self-care of colostomy 1 month after surgery.
> Adequate (as reported by the patient) control of pain during terminal illness and death.
> For the reader of this book: Utilization of the nursing process to assess, plan, implement, and evaluate the care of patients, following graduation from a school of nursing.

Guidelines for Writing All Goal Statements

As you begin to write goal statements for your nursing diagnoses, make sure your long- and short-term goals meet the following criteria:

1. **The goal statement is a patient behavior that demonstrates reduction or alleviation of the problem identified in the nursing diagnosis.** Start with the nursing diagnosis. What is the problem? If the nursing diagnosis is "pain related to broken right arm," the goal will demonstrate alleviation or lessening of the pain. If the nursing diagnosis is "fear of being unable to breast-feed baby related to previous failure with first child," the goal will involve alleviating or lessening the patient's fear of failing at breast-feeding. If the nursing diagnosis is "alterations in bowel elimination," the goal deals with bowel elimination patterns and reestablishing normal function, if possible.

2. **The goal is realistic for the patient's capabilities in the time span you designate in your goal.** A goal for a preterm baby, weighing 4 pounds, that stated, "Baby will weigh 8 pounds at

the end of 1 week," would be unrealistic for this newborn. But if the goal stated, "Baby will weigh 4½ pounds in 7 days," the capabilities of the patient have been considered and make the goal more realistic and more likely to be achieved. Experience, professional literature, references, and advice from other more experienced nurses will help the student learn what is realistic for patients with particular problems.

3. **The goal is realistic for the nurse's level of skill and experience.** If the nursing diagnosis is dealing with a problem beyond the nurse's role, the best course of action is to refer the problem to the appropriate professional. A patient with a nursing diagnosis of "malnutrition related to refusal to eat hospital food" is referred to a dietitian. A patient with a nursing diagnosis of "inability to speak related to recent stroke" is referred to a speech therapist when the patient's condition is sufficiently stable.

4. **The goal is congruent with and supportive of other therapies.** This means that nursing goals for the patient do not contradict or interfere with the work of other professionals caring for the patient. If the nursing diagnosis is "muscle weakness related to bedrest" and the physician has ordered bedrest for 2 more weeks, a nursing goal involving getting the patient out of bed would contradict the medical order and be inappropriate.

5. **Whenever possible the goal is important and valued by the patient, the nurses, and the physician.** If the goals are important to the patients, they will be more motivated to reach a goal. If nurses value the goal, they will be more likely to carry out the suggested plan of care. The physician's understanding and support of nursing goals will help to assure congruence with medical treatment. The goals also serve as a communication tool that keeps health team members informed of the patient's progress.

6. **Write goals in observable or measurable terms whenever possible.** Try to avoid words such as good, normal, adequate, and improved. These words means different things to different people and tend to make the goal unclear. There may be disagreement as to whether the goal was achieved if words requiring a judgment are used in the goal statement.

Observable Goal	Vague Goal
The patient will walk the length of the hall unassisted by 2/5.	Increased ambulation or adequate leg strength
Patient will gain 1/4 lb each week until discharged.	Increased intake or good nutrition or promote weight gain

7.   Write goals in terms of patient outcomes, not nursing actions.

Patient Outcomes	Nursing Actions
The patient will void by 6 P.M.	I will offer the patient the urinal every 2 hours.
The patient will bathe her baby before she is discharged.	I will show the patient a baby bath before she is discharged.
The patient's temperature will be up to 98°F within 1 hour.	I will put warm blankets and a heating pad on the patient and recheck his temperature in 1 hour.

8.   Keep the goal short.
9.   Make the goal specific.
10. Derive each goal from only one nursing diagnosis.
11. Designate a specific time for achievement of each goal.

Goal Statement (Long or Short Term) = Patient Behavior + Criteria of Performance + Time + Conditions (if Needed)

PATIENT BEHAVIOR = an observable activity that the patient will demonstrate
—(the patient) will void
—decrease in (the patient's) blood pressure
—(the patient) will ambulate
—(the patient) will report
—(the patient) will drink

The word "patient" or the patient's actual name may be omitted when writing the goal, since the goal always refers to the patient.

CRITERIA OF ACCEPTABLE PERFORMANCE = the level at which the patient will perform the behavior. How well? How long? How far? How much? A long-term goal attempts to describe the optimum level of eventual functioning.

—At least 500 ml

—below the value of 160/100mm Hg

—the length of the hall, three times

—adequacy of pain management techniques

—1500 ml of liquids

TIME = the designated time or date when the patient should be able to achieve the behavior. A long-term goal attempts to identify how long it will take a patient to achieve the optimal functioning described in the criteria above.

—within the next hour

—by discharge

—at the end of this shift

—by June 5

CONDITION = the circumstances, if important, under which the behavior will be performed. All goals will not have a condition. If the condition is important, put it in the goal statement; if it is not important, leave it out.

—with the help of a walker

—with the use of a wheelchair

—with the help of the family

—with the use of medications

The following examples combine these elements to form goal statements.

Patient Behavior	+	Criteria	+	Time + Condition (if relevant) = GOAL

Patient Behavior	Criteria	Time + Condition
Weight gain	of ½ ounce	every day until discharge.
Weight gain	of ¼ ounce	every day until discharge, . . . on breastfeeding.
Self-injection of insulin	using sterile technique	by November 4.
Maintenance of joint mobility	at current level	while on bedrest.
Regain	birthweight	by 2 weeks of age.
Oral intake	of 500 ml	by 3 p.m. . . . without abdominal distention.

The following examples in Table 2–1 demonstrate the relationship between the nursing diagnosis and the goal statement. A general diagnosis and goal is presented with individualized patient examples.

Table 2–1

Nursing Diagnoses	Goal Statements
Alterations in bowel elimination: Constipation	Reestablish normal bowel patterns (long-term goal)
—alteration in bowel elimination: constipation related to dehydration and inadequate nutritional intake	—bowel movement by 3 P.M. today (short-term goal)
—alteration in bowel elimination: constipation related to bedrest	—bowel movement at least every third day, which is soft and easy to pass (short-term goal)
Knowledge deficit	Possession of knowledge in deficit area (long-term goal)
—knowledge deficit related to diabetic nutritional requirements	—(patient will) plan a 3-day menu that meets diabetic nutritional requirements by June 7 (short-term goal)
—knowledge deficit related to infant care	—(parents) to describe formula preparation and feeding schedule to meet newborn nutritional needs by discharge (short-term goal)
—knowledge deficit related to self-care of colostomy	—(patient) to describe activities involved in caring for colostomy at home by August 15 (short-term goal)
Alterations in comfort	Reestablish comfort (long-term goal)
—alteration in comfort: incisional pain related to surgery	—report of adequate pain management during hospitalization (short-term goal)

Some goals are designed to maintain a continuous level of functioning during the time the patient is receiving nursing care. These goals do not have a specified time for goal achievement but rather imply systematic assessment and evaluation for as long as the problem exists. These goals are considered long-term goals and span several days to weeks or more. For example:

1. Patient to report pain management techniques are adequate during hospitalization.

2. Patient to report pain remains below 4 on a 1–10 scale during the postoperative period.
3. Skin integrity maintained during hospitalization.
4. Normal breath sounds maintained during postoperative period.
5. Maintenance of body weight between 135 and 140 pounds (forever).

These goals would be evaluated periodically as part of the plan of care rather than having a set time or date for evaluation as with other goals discussed. For example (see goals above):

1. Assess pain every 3 to 4 hours
2. Assess pain on 1–10 scale every 3 to 4 hours
3. Assess skin integrity every 2 hours
4. Assess breath sounds every 4 hours
5. Assess body weight every morning

These assessments would then be documented in the patient's chart until the problem or the potential for the problem was resolved.

Practice Exercise

Pick out the correctly written goal statements. Identify what is wrong with the incorrectly written goals. The answers are on the following page.

1. The patient's hydration will improve.
2. The nurse will reduce the patient's anxiety.
3. The patient will know about infant feeding.
4. Improve muscle strength.
5. 3/5: The patient will lose 6 lb in 2 weeks.
6. The patient will talk about her labor within 24 hours after delivery.
7. The decubitus ulcer (bedsore) will be healed by 2/5.
8. Verbalization of decreased pain within the next hour.
9. The patient will express confidence in her ability to breast-feed her baby before discharge.
10. Turn and deep breathe the patient every 2 hours.
11. Ankle edema will decrease.
12. The patient will feel better by bedtime.
13. The patient will ambulate.

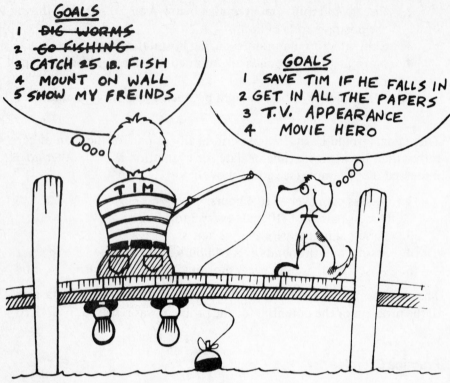

FIGURE 2–2. Goal setting.

14. Teach the patient AROM (active range of motion) exercises.
15. The patient's depression will improve.
16. The patient will learn about good nutrition.
17. The patient will understand the purpose of his medications before discharge.
18. The patient's temperature will stay below 101°F during the next 24 hours.
19. The nursing student will understand the nursing process after reading this book.
20. The student will write a nursing diagnosis and a goal after finishing this chapter.

Answers to Exercise on Goal Statements

1. Not specific or observable. A better goal would be:
   The patient's intake will be 2500 cc every 24 hours.
   or
   The patient will drink at least 75 cc each hour.

2. Not observable. This is a nurse behavior instead of patient behavior. No time limit is set. A better goal would be:
Verbalization of reduced anxiety about tomorrow's surgery by 10 P.M. tonight.
or
The patient will discuss feelings related to biopsy by 3 P.M. today.

3. Not observable, no time limit. A better goal would be:
(The patient) Feeding her baby the majority of his feedings by 6/7.
or
Newborn regained birth weight on breast milk by 2-week checkup.

4. No subject, not specific, no criteria. A better goal would be:
The patient will lift his own weight using the bed trapeze by 2/5.
or
4/5 The patient will be able to lift equal amounts of weight in 3 months with his right and his left arm.

5. O.K.

6. O.K.

7. O.K.

8. O.K. Subject (the patient) is assumed.

9. O.K.

10. This is a nursing action, not an observable patient behavior.

11. Not specific, no time limit. A better goal would be:
Absence of pitting edema of the ankle by tomorrow at 10 P.M.
or
Ankle will measure less than 11 inches in circumference by tomorrow at 8 A.M.

12. Not observable. A better goal would be:
The patient will state she feels better by 10 P.M.

13. No criteria. A better goal would be:
The patient will walk the length of the hall by date of discharge without use of a walker.
or
8/2: The patient will walk from his bed to a chair in his room by tomorrow.

14. Nursing action instead of patient behavior, no time limit. A better goal would be:
The patient will demonstrate AROM by 3 P.M. today.
or

The patient will have equal motion in the right and left shoulder joint by time of discharge.

15. Too vague, not observable. A better goal would be:

The patient will sit in patient lounge for 15 minutes during this shift.

or

8/3: The patient will get dressed and comb her hair tomorrow A.M.

16. Not observable. A better goal would be:

(The patient) Select a food from each of the four basic food groups for tonight's supper.

or

(The patient) Plan a week's menus for a low-salt diet with the help of the dietitian before discharge.

17. Not observable. A better goal would be:

The patient will state the purpose of each of his medications before discharge.

or

By 4/7, the patient will state route, dose, and time for each take-home medication.

18. O.K.

19. Not observable. A better goal would be:

The nursing student will list the steps in the nursing process after reading this book.

or

The nursing student will write one nursing care plan after reading this book.

20. O.K.

PLANNING NURSING INTERVENTIONS

Nursing interventions are activities the nurse plans and implements to help a patient achieve identified goals. By achieving these goals, the patient will reduce or eliminate the problems diagnosed during the assessment phase of the nursing process. Nursing interventions may be referred to in several ways, including nursing actions, nursing strategies, nursing treatment plans, and nursing orders. The nurse, using a problem-solving approach, selects activities to do with and for the patient that are most likely to result in goal achievement.

The planned nursing interventions are communicated to other nurses on the patient care plan to promote a consistent approach toward goal achievement. Often the nurse who has the most information about the patient and expertise in the particular problem areas diagnosed is the one who selects the most appropriate nursing interventions. The written care plan communicates this plan for goal achievement to others who will provide 24-hour nursing care to the patient. The nursing interventions written on the patient's care plan are instructions for others to follow since they may not have the knowledge of or experience with the patient that the original nurse gained during the assessment phase.

Nursing interventions are similar to physician's orders since they specify a plan of care aimed at achieving a goal. In order for others to follow a plan of care, it must be specific or the plan may be interpreted inappropriately. Interventions should identify:

—what is to be done
—when the activity is to be done; how often
—the duration for each intervention, when appropriate
—any preceding or follow-up activities
—the date interventions were selected
—the sequence in which nursing activities are to be performed, when one activity is dependent on or facilitated by a previous action.
—signature or initials of the nurse writing the plan of care

When these things are identified on a patient's plan of nursing care, a nurse is held responsible and accountable for the prescribed care. Other nurses know to whom to direct questions regarding the patient. They know to whom to direct feedback regarding patient responses following the prescribed care. Physicians may seek out the nurse who wrote the plan of care for a patient as the person most knowledgeable about that patient's response to ordered treatments. All of this may seem somewhat threatening to the student in nursing who may feel unsure of abilities to identify accurate diagnoses, select appropriate goals, and choose nursing interventions most likely to achieve those goals. It is a learning process, but without both positive and negative feedback from other nurses who carry out your plan, you will not improve your skills in planning patient care.

NURSING INTERVENTIONS:

Those specific activities the nurse plans and implements in order to help the patient achieve a goal.

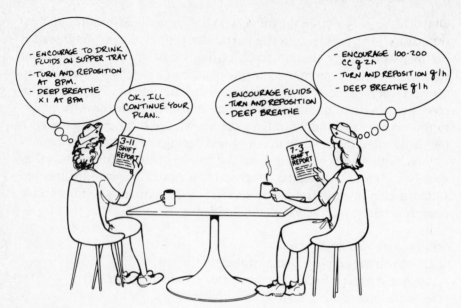

FIGURE 2–3.   Care plans ensure continuity of care.

Some examples of nursing interventions are the following:

SHORT-TERM GOAL: Reestablish urinary elimination, with complete emptying of the bladder within 8 hours of removal of catheter.

—Interventions:

1. Offer assistance to the bathroom for voiding every 2 hours
2. Encourage fluids, 1 glass of juice, every hour
3. Record intake and output for 24 hours
4. Offer analgesics every 3 to 4 hours
5. Encourage voiding attempt in sitz bath, tub bath, or shower if unable to void in 6 hours
6. Provide privacy for voiding attempts
7. Run water in bathroom for voiding attempts
8. Encourage application of pressure over bladder during voiding attempts.
9. Assess bladder for emptying following voiding

12/6 3ᴾᴹ L. Atkinson R.N.

Nursing actions are based on principles and knowledge integrated from previous nursing education and experience and from the behavioral and physical sciences. These principles identify the proven relationship between the nursing intervention and goal achievement. Nursing actions are known to affect people in predictable ways and are chosen to help a patient achieve a goal because of these expected outcomes. For example, the effects of heat and cold applied to the skin are understood by the nurse. If the nurse wants to increase the blood flow to an area of the body as one way of promoting goal achievement, a nursing intervention such as "warm packs to right arm, 20 minutes 4 times a day" might be chosen.

The first courses in many nursing programs involve the student in a study of basic fundamentals of nursing practice. These fundamentals courses provide the student with the rationale for the steps of various skills and procedures in addition to teaching the motor aspects of the skill or procedure. In order to safely adapt nursing care to new situations, new equipment, and changing technology, the nurse must understand the rationale behind the choice of nursing actions. Principles and theories related to sterile technique, for example, have remained constant as equipment and materials changed from reusable supplies to disposable. The nurse who understands the rationale behind sterile technique for various procedures is more able to adapt nursing care to a particular patient using any variety of equipment and supplies available. Principles and theories from disciplines related to nursing, such as anatomy, physiology, psychology, and sociology, blend with nursing knowledge and experience to form an integrated base of knowledge that guides the nurse in planning patient care. While the nursing process involves an understanding of the rationale underlying nursing actions, it is not necessary to include this written rationale in documenting the care plan. However, the nursing process is incomplete and potentially unsafe unless nurses base their choices of nursing actions on appropriate rationale. Rationale for nursing actions are included in the various care plans in this text as a teaching tool. In clinical settings, writing rationale for nursing actions consumes much time and space and therefore is inappropriate.

The following example illustrates the principles and theories from various disciplines upon which selection of appropriate nursing actions are based.

NURSING DIAGNOSIS: Pain related to cervical dilatation of labor. (Alterations in comfort: Pain related to L & D)

NURSING GOAL: Patient verbalizations related to adequate pain relief measures during labor.

Nursing Interventions	*Rationale*
a. Encourage husband to stay with wife, if desired by the couple.	a. When individuals are under stress, presence of their support system can reduce the effects of stress.
b. Assess q½-1h for signs of muscle tension. Encourage relaxation through massage, heat, cold, and slow breathing when possible.	b. Fear can lead to increased muscle tension. Increased muscle tension can lead to increased perception of pain. Continuous muscle tension depletes energy reserves. Massage of tense muscles may help individuals to relax those muscles. Heat or cold may feel soothing as labor progresses and aid relaxation. Muscle tension can be reduced as patients consciously relax while slowly exhaling.
c. Keep couple informed of progress. Encourage questions; explanations.	c. Fear may be caused by insufficient or inaccurate information.
d. Assist with breathing techniques learned for labor.	d. Individuals can be conditioned to respond to a stimulus with specific learned behavior. Distraction can help lessen pain perception. Practice with feedback leads to improved performance.
e. Encourage use of a focal point.	e. Visual concentration may distract from pain perception.
f. Offer technique of effleurage.	f. Tactile stimulation can interfere with deeper pain sensations.
g. Verbal encouragement and praise for efforts to manage discomfort of labor.	g. Positive reinforcement of desired behavior increases the occurrence of that behavior.
h. Request order for analgesics p.r.n.; assess need qh	h. Chemical agents alter the perception of pain.
i. Assess cervical dilatation and fetal heart rate before administering any analgesics.	i. Analgesics given late in labor may depress the fetus at birth. Cervical dilatation may change rapidly in the active phase of labor. Fetal heart rate is an indicator of fetal well-being. Analgesics given to the mother can further depress a compromised fetus.

3/7 L. Atkinson R.N.

Problem Solving and Selecting Interventions

How does a nurse choose the most appropriate interventions? Some nurses just seem to to "know" what to do to help a patient achieve a goal. Others do things because "we have always done it this way." Still others rely on a standard care plan designed for all patients with similar problems to tell them what to do. Where does a student begin? Nursing is not based on intuition. You have to learn how to be an effective nurse. That means applying the skills of problem solving to a particular patient's health problems and the environment in which nursing care is to be given. The following steps may be helpful to you as you develop a plan of care for a patient:

1. Review the nursing diagnosis and the priorities you set among them.
2. Examine the goal so you have a clear picture of your desired outcomes.
3. Consider all possible nursing activities that might help the patient achieve the goal:
   —changes in the environment
   —activities for the patient to perform independently
   —activities to perform with the patient
   —activities to perform for the patient
   —assistance from other health professionals
   —involvement of the patient's friends and family
   —changes in the nurse (increased knowledge and skill)

   Use standards of patient care as guidelines for developing and planning a patient's nursing care. Standards of patient care may be available to you on index cards that will fit in a Kardex care plan. These standards provide the nurse with general guidelines for patients with particular medical diagnoses, diagnostic studies, or nursing diagnoses. They identify areas for assessment, possible patient problems to anticipate, and suggested nursing interventions. They provide the student and the nurse with another resource for planning nursing interventions. These standards of care do not replace the individualized care plan developed by the nurse following the assessment phase. Based on the knowledge about an individual patient, the medical management of health problems, the health care setting, and patient and family preferences and concerns, the nurse will delete inappropriate interventions, add new inter-

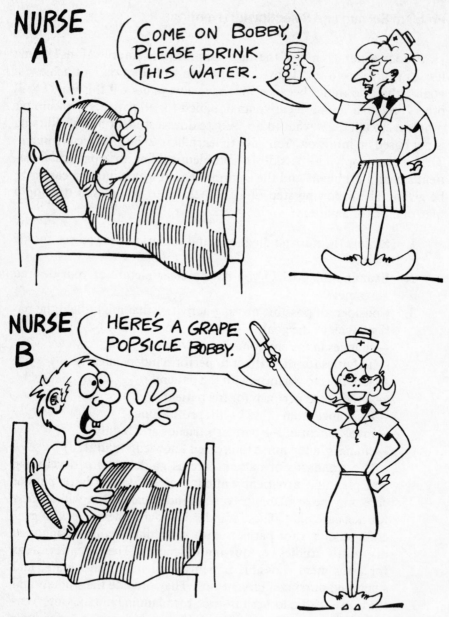

FIGURE 2–4. Whenever possible, nursing actions should take the patient's preferences into account.

ventions, and modify and clarify general interventions. These plans save the nurse time in rewriting common nursing interventions but do not replace the process of planning individualized care.

Use the patient and the patient's family as a source of possible nursing interventions. Patients may have many good suggestions for activities they can perform, with or without nursing assistance, to achieve a certain goal, based on their past experiences and personal preferences. The nurse then uses personal knowledge and experience to incorporate some of the patient's suggestions into a plan of care. This collaboration helps to involve patients in planning and implementing the type of nursing care they receive. By using the patient and family to help plan nursing interventions, the nurse considers patient preferences, which usually leads to more effective interventions.

4. Consider the advantages and disadvantages of possible nursing interventions and select those that meet the following criteria:

- **Nursing actions must be safe for the patient.** Application of heat to the skin will stimulate circulation, but excessive heat will burn. Nursing actions using heat must ensure that the patient is not burned. Exercising a patient's muscles and joints can be very beneficial; however, if muscles and joints are forced beyond the point of resistance or pain, the nurse can cause injuries.

- **Nursing actions must be congruent with other therapies.** For example, nursing actions must be selected within the safety range ordered by the physician. If the medical order reads "Aspirin (ASA), 2 tablets, q4h, prn," nursing actions cannot plan the administration of aspirin every 2 hours. If the physical therapist is instructing the patient in the use of a walker, the nurse should also use a walker in ambulating the patient.

- **Nursing actions selected are most likely to develop the behavior described in the goal statement.** There may be many different nursing actions that would accomplish the same goal. The nurse attempts to give the patient practice in the specific behavior stated in the goal. For example:

  NURSING DIAGNOSIS: Pain related to bone cancer.
  NURSING GOAL: Verbalization related to experiencing minimal pain during hospitalization; less than 3 on a 1–10 scale.

	Nursing Actions/Interventions
May Achieve Goal	*More Likely to Achieve Goal*
a. Offer prescribed pain medication q3–4h	a. Assess patient's pain, timing, duration, intensity, and related activities, q3–4h
	b. Assess patient's current methods of dealing with pain and support as possible
	c. Discuss and practice alternate pain relief measures with patient, by March 1 (1) Relaxation (2) Alternative sensory stimulation —music —tactile (massage, effleurage, menthol rubs, vibrators) —heat/cold —movies, TV, reading (3) Breathing techniques
	d. Discuss self-medication for pain, by March 3
	e. Discuss effectiveness of pain relief measures with physician and patient
	f. Encourage use of pain relief measures when discomfort *begins* rather than after it is intense

2/28 *L. Atkinson R.N.*

- **Nursing actions are realistic:**
  —for the patient. Consider age, physical strength, disease, willingness to change behavior, resources.
  —for the number of hospital staff. Will enough people consistently be available to carry out the nursing actions?
  —for the experience and ability of available staff. If most of the staff are unfamiliar with the nursing actions you are suggesting, there is a high probability they will not be carried out.
  —for available equipment. If your nursing actions include the use of any equipment, it should be readily available and the hospital staff should be familiar with its use.

- **Nursing actions consider meeting lower level survival needs before higher level needs.** For example, the following sequence of nursing actions deals with the current need of pain avoidance before asking the patient to deal with potential problems.

  NURSING DIAGNOSIS: Prone to respiratory complications following surgery with general anesthesia.

  NURSING GOAL: Normal respiratory rate and lung sounds within 24 hours postop.

  NURSING ACTIONS
    a. Explain goal to patient.
    b. Explain preventive function of the following activities.
       (1) Turning, coughing, and deep breathing at least every 2 hours.
       (2) Early ambulation.
       (3) Use of deep-breathing device.
    c. Explain ways to minimize discomfort during turning and coughing; splinting, analgesics.
    d. Offer pain medication 1/2 hour prior to ambulating.
    e. Assist patient to:
       (1) TCH q2 h × 24 h
       (2) Ambulate q.i.d. starting first postop day.
       (3) Deep breath q1 h while awake × 24 h.
    f. Assess lung sounds before and after TCH sessions.

- **Nursing actions needed to assess and monitor effect of medical treatments are included.** Some medical orders may require nursing activities such as patient assessment, prior to carrying out the physician's order, to ensure patient safety. For example:

  MEDICAL ORDER: Lanoxin 0.125 mg qd

  NURSING ACTION:
    a. Count apical pulse *prior* to *every* medication administration.
    b. Give Lanoxin 0.125 mg at 8 A.M. qd if pulse above 60 beats per minute. Hold if pulse significantly above previously recorded rate or below 60 beats per minute.
    c. Notify physician if medication held.

  MEDICAL ORDER: Magnesium sulfate 5 gm deep IM q6 h.

NURSING ACTIONS:
   a. Assess patient's reflexes, urine output, and respira-
      tory rate *prior* to *every* medication administration.
   b. Give $MgSO_4$ 5 gm deep IM at 8A–2P–8P–2A if re-
      flexes normal or brisk. Hold medication and con-
      sult physician if reflexes are depressed or absent; if
      urine output is less than 30 cc per hour, or if respi-
      rations are below 12 breaths per minute.

• **Whenever possible, nursing actions should be important to
  the patient and compatible with personal goals and values.**
  The patient should understand how the nursing actions will
  result in achievement of the goal. For example, a 5-year-old
  boy may not understand the importance of good nutrition
  to his recovery, but he may love to play games. If the nursing actions can make a game out of eating, the child may
  begin to eat more because he values the eating game the
  nurse has created. A man may refuse to do arm and hand
  exercises because he does not think they are important. If
  the nursing actions encourage the patient to do activities
  such as shaving, combing his hair, brushing his teeth, and
  feeding himself, the arms and hands will still receive the
  desired exercise. The difference is that the patient values
  being able to do these self-care activities and can see that
  they are part of his recovery.

Developing a Teaching Plan

If the nurse assesses a patient and makes a nursing diagnosis related to a
knowledge or performance deficit, a teaching plan will most likely comprise a large portion of the activity in the planning phase of the nursing
process. Inadequate or incorrect knowledge may also be related to various other patient problems. Unrealistic fears of a medical procedure
and incorrectly taking prescribed medications are examples of problems
that could be caused by the patient's belief in erroneous information.
Patients with newly diagnosed medical problems are frequently con-
fronted with knowledge deficits concerning the implications of their
medical diagnosis and the effect it may have on their life-style. Patients
taking on new roles, such as parenting, are frequently concerned about
their lack of knowledge and skill in newborn care. Prenatal classes such
as Lamaze and CEA will anticipate these learning needs and identify

specific areas of newborn care that prospective parents would like to discuss in class. Nursing follow-through in the hospital, after delivery, builds on this information and gives the parents actual practice in caring for their newborn. Similarly, preoperative and postoperative teaching is based on a nursing diagnosis related to inadequate knowledge of the surgical experience, complications, and preventive measures. Preoperative teaching is also based on research indicating that an educated patient, knowing what will happen during a procedure, will often experience less pain and anxiety than an unprepared patient. The nursing diagnosis, again, would relate to inadequate or incorrect information about a particular procedure or surgery.

In applying the nursing process to the formulation of a teaching plan, the nurse follows a logical sequence of problem solving. First, the knowledge deficit is identified in the assessment phase of the nursing process. A goal is then chosen that identifies the learning outcomes. Next, a plan is developed to teach the skill or information to the patient.

For example:

1. NURSING DIAGNOSIS: Lack of knowledge and skill in taking newborn rectal temperature.

   GOAL: Take an accurate rectal temperature on her newborn before discharge, on 3/5.

   NURSING INTERVENTIONS (Teaching Plan):

   1. Demonstrate how to take rectal temperatures on newborns, 3/4.
   2. Explain safety precautions and when to notify physician for fevers, 3/4.
   3. Provide reinforced practice in taking her newborn's temperature, 3/4.

2. NURSING DIAGNOSIS: Knowledge deficit related to taking medications.

   GOAL: Demonstrate correct self-administration of medication by 11/3.

   1. Check that patient can read all labels on medications, 11/1.
   2. Discuss with the patient how to safely take each medication (drug, dose, time, route), 11/1.
   3. Provide a clear set of directions in written form regarding medications, 11/1.
   4. Supervise patient in hospital with self-administration of prescribed medications, 11/1, 11/2.

When patients learn specific motor skills, the goal selected has a very direct relationship to the diagnosed knowledge or performance deficit. The teaching plan and eventually the evaluation of the patient's ability to perform the skill are usually equally specific. When teaching motor skills follow the steps of the nursing process:

1. Identify knowledge deficits (NURSING DIAGNOSIS)
   —Inadequate skill related to . . .
   —Knowledge deficit related to performance of . . .
2. Identify the specific behavior the patient will perform based on the diagnosed learning need (GOAL).
3. Teach the specific behavior to the patient (NURSING INTERVENTIONS).
4. Test the patient's ability to perform the specific behavior (EVALUATION).

Evaluating patient learning may be difficult if observable behaviors are not identified as goals during the planning phase. When a patient is developing an understanding of broader concepts or improving cognitive skills, the nurse's teaching plan cannot focus on one specific behavior as evidence of this broader understanding. For example, if the diagnosis relates to inadequate knowledge of infant care, a goal dealing with the isolated behavior of diapering does not provide support for the assumption that the parent is competent in infant care. In this case, the method the nurse may use is the identification of one long-term learning goal and then subsequent identification of several short-term goals that are examples of the long-term goal. The long-term goal may be more difficult to state in behavioral terms. The examples of short-term goals should be stated as observable or measurable behaviors. The teaching plan is then directed at the long-term goal by achieving the short-term goals.

Example 1:

NURSING DIAGNOSIS: Inadequate knowledge and skill related to newborn care.

LONG-TERM GOAL: Parents will safely care for newborn by time of discharge from hospital, on 11/3.

SHORT-TERM GOALS:

1. Demonstrate bathing their newborn, 11/2.
2. Safely take a rectal temperature on newborn, 11/2.
3. Demonstrate cord care for umbilical stump, 11/2.
4. Breast-feeding: 10-15 minutes per breast q 2-5 h, by 11/3.
5. Transport newborn home from hospital in infant car seat, 11/3.

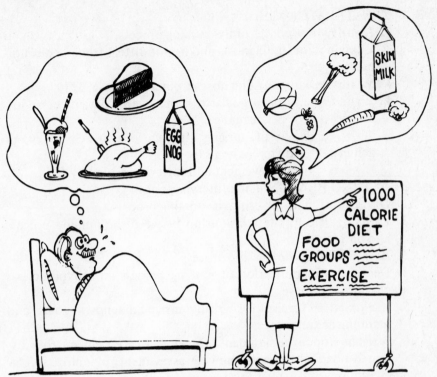

FIGURE 2–5. A good teaching plan does not always guarantee that patient learning will occur.

TEACHING PLAN: Nursing Interventions
1. Assess readiness for learning infant care (comfort level, fatigue, personal priority needs).
2. Discuss various aspects of infant care: feedings, hygiene, safety, growth and development, behavior.
3. Demonstrate specific infant care skills and provide practice for parents with positive reinforcement.
4. Assist in initiation of breast-feeding and provide specific information on the skill.
5. Provide resources for parents after discharge (people to call when questions or problems arise).

Example 2:

NURSING DIAGNOSIS: Inadequate knowledge related to the nursing process.

LONG-TERM GOAL: Student will correctly utilize the nursing process in providing patient care by 6/1.

SHORT-TERM GOALS:
1. Identify four phases of the nursing process, 3/1.
2. Explain nursing diagnosis and how it differs from medical diagnosis, 3/5.
3. Write three nursing diagnoses from a data base, 3/10.
4. Write three nursing goals with observable patient behavior, and criteria of performance, 3/20.
5. Write three sets of nursing interventions to help a patient achieve three different goals by 4/1.
6. Evaluate goal achievement and review care plan by 4/10.

TEACHING PLAN: Nursing Interventions
1. Discuss rationale for using the nursing process.
2. Explain, briefly, the relationship between the nursing process and patient care.
3. Assign readings on nursing process.
4. Demonstrate application of nursing process on a hypothetical patient's database.
5. Use practice exercises for writing nursing diagnoses, goals, and planning actions.
6. Written student assignment: Develop a care plan on four assigned hospital patients showing assessment, planning, implementation, and evaluation.
7. Review and critique other students' care plans.

There are several things to consider when developing a teaching plan. Learning is enhanced by using principles of teaching-learning. It is especially important to assess the patient's readiness to learn. An illness, medical problem, or treatment may greatly interfere with learning, particularly in the acute phase of an illness. Medications, fatigue, motivation, anxiety, pain, or hunger may all block effective learning. Teaching should be delayed until some of these obstacles have been lessened or eliminated. The nurse also assesses the patient's previous knowledge and skills, building on this prior base. Begin at the level of patient understanding using language understandable to the patient. Individualizing the teaching approach may also lead to improved patient learning. The following principles support these common nursing interventions as part of a teaching plan.

Common Components of a Teaching Plan	Rationale and Scientific Principles
1. Setting a learning goal with the patient.	1. Clarification of desired learning outcomes will guide teaching methods and may serve as a motivating function for the learner.
2. Assessing patient's readiness to learn. 　a. motivation-recognizes knowledge deficit 　b. illness/medical problem 　c. medication/pain 　d. level of consciousness 　e. anxiety level 　f. fatigue	2. A person learns more effectively when the learning experience has personal relevance. A person learns more effectively when a need to learn is perceived. Unmet physical or psychosocial needs such as anxiety, pain, and fatigue have a negative effect on attention, retention, and ability to learn.
3. Assess patient's current knowledge and motor skill ability. 4. Begin teaching at the patient's current level of understanding or skill performance.	3., 4. Teaching that moves from simple to complex will help to ensure understanding. Simple and complex are relative terms and have meaning only in relationship to the learner's current level of understanding or performance.
5. Provide the patient with an opportunity to practice motor skills after a demonstration. 6. Reinforce patient's efforts to learn whenever possible.	5., 6. An active learner learns and retains more than a passive learner. Practice with feedback and positive reinforcement leads to improved performance and continuance of reinforced behavior.

The care plan for Mrs. Witten follows. The database and nursing diagnoses were developed in Chapter 1. Chapter 3 contains an abbreviated form of the total plan as it might appear on a nursing Kardex. Chapter 4 contains an evaluation of the plan.

NURSING CARE PLAN FOR MRS. WITTEN

Diagnoses

Alteration in comfort: acute pain related to probable gallbladder disease (high priority)

Goals

Patient to report pain management techniques adequate preoperatively

Interventions

1. Assess what activities precipitate/intensify pain and avoid. Encourage activities patient employs to reduce pain if safe.
2. Assess pain q3h; offer ordered analgesics q3h.
3. Aqua-K heating pad to abdomen as patient desires.
4. Assist with positioning q2h.

Fear related to uncertain outcome and hospitalization (high priority)

Patient to state feeling less fearful of hospital and illness prior to surgery

1. Interventions for pain.
2. Assess understanding of illness and treatment and provide information, prn.
3. Orient to room, equipment, schedules for next 3–4h.
4. Encourage husband to stay.
5. Assign same nurses to care.
6. Encourage verbalization of fears.
7. Answer call light promptly.
8. Assess status q1–2h.

| Knowledge deficit: insufficient knowledge related to surgical treatment (middle priority) | Patient will verbalize course of events for surgery and activities to prevent postop problems within 24h | 1. Assess understanding of information from M.D. and reinforce.
2. Discuss preop, surgical, and postop experience with patient and husband.
3. Discuss pain management and common physical sensations related to surgery.
4. Provide printed information on gallbladder surgery (cholecystectomy).
5. Provide opportunity for questions several hours before surgery. |
| Health maintenance deficit: inability to perform breast self-exam related to lack of information (low priority) | Demonstrate breast self-exam before discharge | 1. Explain importance of early detection and treatment.
2. Timing of exam—q month 1–2 days after menstrual period.
3. Demonstrate exam on pt.
4. Identify abnormal findings to report to M.D. immediately.
5. Provide printed information on breast exam. |

Developed: 6/3/86 L. Atkinson R.N.

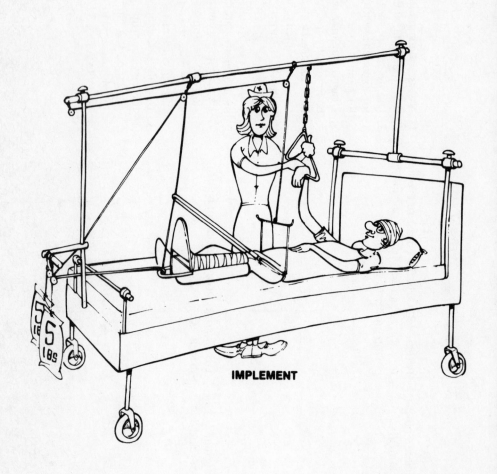

IMPLEMENT

CHAPTER 3

Implementation

Like the other steps comprising the nursing process, the implementation phase consists of several activities: validating the care plan, writing the care plan, giving and documenting nursing care, and continuing to collect data.

$$\text{Implementation} = \frac{\text{Validating}}{\text{Care Plan}} + \frac{\text{Documenting}}{\text{Care Plan}} + \frac{\text{Giving and}}{\text{Documenting}} + \frac{\text{Continuing}}{\text{Data}}$$

Implementation = Validating Care Plan + Documenting Care Plan + Giving and Documenting Nursing Care + Continuing Data Collection

VALIDATING THE CARE PLAN

When nursing students or inexperienced staff nurses write a care plan, it is recommended that they take the proposed care plans to a colleague and request validation. This step does not have to involve a lengthy scheduled consultation but is, rather, a very brief time during which nurses seek the opinion of other nurses. It is important that the student seek appropriate sources for validation. For example, the student may request the clinical instructor or team leader to review the care plan. Such qualified sources can evaluate the care plan by using the following questions as guides.

1. Does the plan assure the patient's safety?
2. Is the plan based on sound scientific principles?
3. Is the plan supported by accepted nursing knowledge?

4. Are the nursing diagnoses supported by the data?
5. Do priorities consider patient desires, physical and psychosocial needs?
6. Does the goal relate to the problem identified in the nursing diagnosis?
7. Does the goal contain a time and patient behavior for evaluation?
8. Can the planned nursing actions realistically assist the patient to achieve the intended goal?
9. Are the nursing actions arranged in a logical sequence?
10. Is the plan individualized to the needs and capabilities of this particular patient?

Thus, the nurse who provides the validation is reviewing the plan in three major areas:

1. Safety
2. Sound nursing practice
3. Individualized nursing care

Because of their expertise in nursing care, other nurses are the most frequently used validating professionals. At times, a nurse may wish to utilize another health team member to review some aspect of a nursing care plan. For example, the nurse teaching a diabetic client about a diabetic exchange diet may wish to have a dietitian validate food substitutions requested by the patient.

Occasionally, a nursing student may select an inappropriate person to validate a care plan. Frequently, nurse aides are very knowledgeable about a specific type of care, having had several years' experience in a particular clinical area. However, the nursing student should not ask aides to validate a care plan. Nurse's aides may be a source for data in that they may be able to provide information about routines of the clinical area, but the nurse aide is not a planner of nursing care. This is a function of the nurse.

Having reviewed the plan with another professional, the student or nurse may wish to share the completed plan with the patient, who is another possible source for validation. The patient can advise the nurse if any aspect of the plan is unacceptable. Not all goals and plans are shared by nurses and patients, but agreement is desirable whenever possible. This gives patients another opportunity to participate in planning their own care. In summary, to validate the plan is to request another appropriate professional and the patient, if possible, to give the plan approval for implementation.

DOCUMENTING THE NURSING CARE PLAN

To retain a nursing care plan for the exclusive use of one nurse is to defeat a primary purpose of care plans. In order to get the maximum effect, a care plan must get the maximum press!

A nurse may plan a patient care conference as a "press conference" for a completed care plan. At such a meeting the nurse summarizes data, problems, goals, and planned actions. The nurse spends most of the time focusing on presenting the care plan to the team. At such a time the nurse may also gain new information from team members to add to the care plan. This conference may also be used as a problem solving session during which a nurse may request assistance from colleagues to further develop a care plan.

Another communication tool is the written care plan. In many hospitals, both physicians and nurses utilize a type of documentation known as a problem oriented medical record (POMR). The care plan in such a system then takes the place of SOAP or (SOAPIER) notes. The

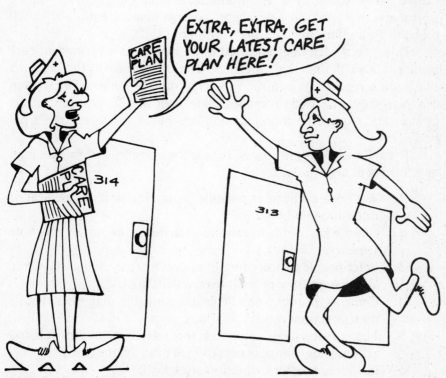

FIGURE 3–1. A nursing care plan must be shared, in order to be effective.

word SOAP is used as an acronym for subjective data, objective data, assessment, and plan. Some formats add the use of the letters IER to include implementation, evaluation, and reassessment.

Other hospitals use a nursing Kardex as a system of organizing care plans. A nursing Kardex is a file that contains the nursing care plans. Each plan is recorded on an oversized index card or large folded sheet of paper. Kardex forms may include space for medical treatments, diagnostic procedures, and other schedules. Still other institutions have adopted 8 1/2 inch × 11 inch nursing care plan forms, which have the advantage of corresponding to standard chart size.

Some computerized hospitals are using the computer to generate a standardized care plan for a patient with a specific diagnosis. (See Care Plan #5 in the appendix.) The nurse begins with this care plan and then modifies it to meet the needs of the individual patient.

The form of the written care plan may vary from institution to institution, but it should be a useful tool for communicating. Most Kardexes will include space for nursing diagnoses, goals, nursing orders, and evaluation in an abbreviated form. A written care plan may be condensed but must convey all essential information. Often nurses will use worksheets to record those problems, goals, and interventions that will probably be accomplished during their 8-hour shift.

This 8-hour plan does not need to be written as a permanent care plan, although the nursing care must be documented in the patient's chart and a report given to the following shift of nurses. The written care plan should be used to communicate goals that cover several shifts or more and require the coordinated efforts of several nurses over a period of time.

The following suggestions will assist the nurse to write a care plan on a Kardex or any similar form.

1. Abbreviate whenever possible, using standardized medical or English symbols.
2. Choose key words to communicate ideas; do not write whole sentences.
3. Refer people to procedure books rather than trying to include all the steps for a procedure on a written plan.
4. Category headings should include nursing diagnoses, goals, nursing actions, and evaluations.
5. The nursing diagnosis with the related goal and nursing actions should appear next to each other on the care plan.
6. Include a date for evaluation of each goal.

7. All long-term goals should be written. Nursing actions directly related to long-term goals should also be written. If a short-term goal will be evaluated within the nurse's 8-hour shift, it is not necessary to include it on the written form. It is necessary to document the nursing care.

8. Short-term goals that cannot be met within an 8-hour shift should be written in order that other nurses can continue the plan of care.

9. Long-term goals being met by a series of short-term goals have both the long-term goals and the progressive short-term goal on the Kardex. The accompanying actions for short-term goals are included. If the short-term goal is to be met during the next few hours by the nurse writing the care plan, the nurse should write the next progressive short-term goal and nursing actions.

10. When goals are evaluated, they should be signed and dated by the responsible nurse.

11. All nursing interventions (actions, orders, or whatever term is being used) should be signed by the registered nurse responsible for writing them.

Table 3-1 shows the nursing care plan for Mrs. Witten as it might appear on a Kardex.

GIVING AND DOCUMENTING NURSING CARE

At last! The nurse now has a plan that will individualize the care given to a patient. Now the nurse is ready to give the care as planned. Even though the nurse has developed an excellent care plan, occasionally (and in the hospital it seems to be the rule), situations occur that interfere with implementing the plan. The patient may be scheduled for emergency surgery. A patient may be in great pain, which alters priorities. Visitors may arrive and the patient is eager to spend time with them. In each case the nurse may be unable to implement the care plan without making some modifications.

Finally, as a last step in implementation, the nurse documents the care given to patients. The nurse is guided by the old maxim "If it is not recorded, it has not been done." If evidence of implementation does not exist in the patient's permanent record, it would seem that the plan has not been followed and the efforts of the nurse have been wasted. In

Table 3–1 Abbreviated Care Plan for Mrs. Witten

Nursing Diagnoses	Goals	Interventions	Evaluation
Know. deficit: insuf. know. r/t surgical tx	Pt. state events r/t surgery and activ. to prevent postop prob. in next 24h	1. Assess understanding of info. from M.D. and reinforce 2. Discuss preop, OR, and postop exp. with family 3. Discuss pain mgmt., common physical sensations 4. Give printed info., chole. 5. Return for quest. 2–3h b/4 surgery	
Health maint. deficit: inability to do SBE r/t lack of information	Demo. SBE before discharge	1. Explain impt. of early detec. and tx 2. Timing of SBE q month 1–2 days after menstru. 3. Demo. of exam for pt. 4. ID abnor. findings to report stat to MD 5. Give printed info on SBE	

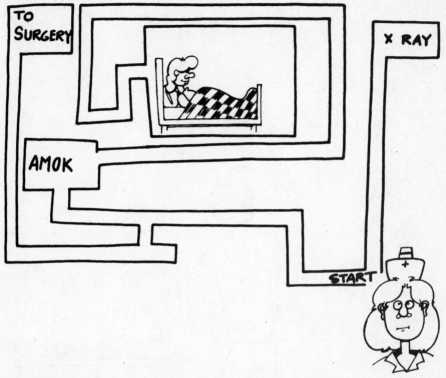

FIGURE 3–2. Even the best laid plans sometimes run amok.

addition, following the nursing interventions planned by a colleague is a way that nurses support each other in developing accountability for nursing care. Few nurses would omit giving or documenting a medication ordered by a physician. The implementation of nursing interventions is equally important to the well-being of patients and thus deserves to be treated seriously, respectfully, and with full accountability.

CONTINUING DATA COLLECTION

Throughout the process of implementation the nurse continues to collect data. As the patient's condition changes, the database changes, subsequently requiring revising and updating of the care plan. Data gathered while giving nursing care may also be used as evidence for evaluation of goal achievement, which will be discussed in the next chapter.

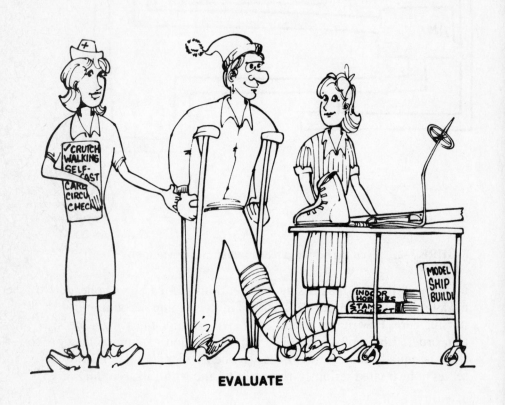

EVALUATE

CHAPTER 4

Evaluation

Evaluation is the last chapter and the final step in the nursing process, yet like the other steps, it is an ongoing activity. There are two parts to evaluation: evaluation of goal achievement and review of the nursing process.

Evaluation	=	Evaluation of Goal Achievement	+	Review of the Nursing Process

EVALUATION OF GOAL ACHIEVEMENT

The purpose of the first part of evaluation is to decide whether the patient has achieved the goal selected during the planning phase of the nursing process. The goal is evaluated at the time or date specified in the goal statement. While giving patient care, the nurse is continuously collecting new data about the patient. Some of this information will be used for evaluation of goal achievement. When evaluating goal achievement, the nurse returns to the goal statement in the care plan. What was the specific patient behavior stated in the goal? Was the patient able to perform the behavior by the time allowed in the goal statement? Was the patient able to perform the behavior as well as described in the criteria part of the goal statement? The answers to these questions are the basis for an evaluation of goal achievement.

The only thing that is evaluated is the patient's ability to demonstrate the behavior described in the goal statement. Nursing actions are not evaluated at this point and are not part of the evaluation statement.

Effectiveness of the nursing actions and teaching plans will be examined during review of the nursing process. The nurse may have given the world's fastest bedbath, but that is not important for evaluating goal achievement. If the goal was to have the patient relax and sleep for several hours, the nurse evaluates the patient's behavior. Did the patient sleep for several hours? The skill with which a nurse performs various procedures is important and will affect goal achievement. However, when an evaluative statement is written, it is the patient's behavior that is assessed. *The outcome of nursing care in the form of changed patient behavior is the focus of goal evaluation.*

Writing an Evaluative Statement

There are two parts to an evaluative statement: a decision on how well the goal was achieved, and the patient data or behavior that supports this decision. The nurse has three alternatives when deciding how well a goal was met: (1) goal met, (2) goal partially met, and (3) goal not met.

If the patient was able to demonstrate the behavior by the specific time or date in the goal statement, the goal was met. If the patient was able to demonstrate the behavior but not as well as the nurse had specified in the goal statement, the goal was partially met. If the patient was unable or unwilling to perform the behavior at all, the goal was not met.

Goal Met
Evaluative Statement = Goal Partially Met + Actual Patient Behavior as Evidence
Goal Not Met

In the evaluative statement, the nurse includes a description of the patient's actual behavior as the individual tries to demonstrate the behavior identified in the goal. For example, if the behavior identified in the goal was for the patient to report some degree of pain relief, the nurse talks with the patient regarding severity of pain, following the nursing interventions to help relieve it. The patient's response about the severity of current pain makes up the second part of the evaluative statement.

For example:

1. **Goal Statement:** Patient will walk length of hall and back by 2/7.
    Goal Evaluation (done on 2/7 or earlier):
    Goal achieved; patient walked length of hall and back.

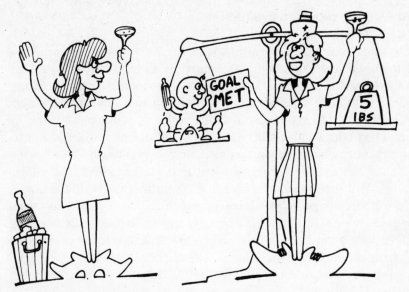

FIGURE 4–1. Goal met—congratulations!

Goal partially achieved; patient walked length of hall but too tired to walk back.

Goal not achieved; patient refused to walk.

Goal not achieved; patient unable to bear his own weight.

2. **Goal Statement:** 2/7 Decubitus ulcer (bedsore) will be healed in 1 month.

Goal Evaluation (done on 3/7 or earlier):

Goal met; decubitus ulcer healed.

Goal partially met; decubitus ulcer still present but is 1/2 the size and dry.

Goal not met; decubitus ulcer broken open and draining.

3. **Goal Statement:** After finishing Chapter 4, the student will state this nursing process book is the most interesting book ever read.

Goal Evaluation (done when the student finishes Chapter 4):

Goal met; student stated this book was the most interesting book ever read and asked for an *A* in the course.

Goal partially met; student said this book was about as interesting as any other course books, and asked for a *C* in the course.

Goal not met; student lost book and asked for a class withdrawal slip.

Patient Participation and Evaluation

Evaluation of goal achievement is done with the patient whenever possible. It may also be done with the patient's family. It is not just the nurse's assessment of the patient's ability to achieve a goal that is important. The patient's perception is also important since the problem identified in the nursing diagnosis is the patient's problem and not the nurse's. The patient who evaluates personal goal achievement is a partner with the nurse and receives feedback on progress toward eliminating or reducing the original problem identified in the assessment phase. When a patient successfully achieves a goal mutually set with the nurse, that person receives positive reinforcement to continue efforts toward a higher level of functioning. This concept of evaluating goals with the patient is spelled out in one of the eight standards of nursing practice of the American Nurses' Association: "The client's/patient's progress or lack of progress toward goal achievement is determined by the client/patient and the nurse."

When evaluating goal achievement, the nurse is responsible for documenting both parts of the goal statement. This may be done in the patient's chart. The care plan on the Kardex will also include this evaluation. The nurse doing the evaluation with the patient includes the date the evaluation was done, whether or not the goal was achieved, subjective and objective data related to the patient's behavior compared to the behavior identified in the goal, and the nurse's signature. For example:

Goals	Evaluation
1. Understanding of self-care needs associated with diabetes as evidenced by performing the following before discharge: a. Short-term: Planning a 3-day menu for family that meets diabetic diet requirements. Long-term: Prevention of severe hyperglycemia (4 + urine glucose or 2%) after discharge from hospital.	a. Short-term: Goal met 11/13. Dietitian reported patient able to plan 3-day menu meeting diabetic diet requirements. Long-term: Goal not evaluated. Referred to public health nurse for follow-up visits. *L. Atkinson RN.*
b. Listing signs and symptoms of hyperglycemia and hypoglycemia.	b. Goal partially met 11/15. Patient lists hypoglycemia signs and symptoms. Confused on hyperglycemia. *L. Atkinson RN.*

Goals	*Evaluation*
Explaining actions to take for hyperglycemia and hypoglycemia.	Goal met. Patient stated appropriate actions to deal with hyperglycemia and hypoglycemia 11/12. *L. atkinson R.N.*
c. Correctly performing diabetic urine testing.	c. Goal met. Correctly tested urine qid × 2 d, 11/13–14. *L. atkinson R.N.*
d. Correctly performing diabetic foot care.	d. Goal met. Performed foot care correctly × 2. 11/14. *L. atkinson R.N.*
e. Absence of skin infections during hospitaliztion and after discharge; demonstrating diabetic skin care.	e. Goal partially met. No skin infections occurred during hospitalization. Referred to public health nurse for follow-up visits. Demonstrated appropriate skin care. 11/16. *L. atkinson, R.N.*
f. Demonstrating competence in self-administration of oral hypoglycemic medication.	f. Goal met. Competent self-administration of Diabinase 0.250 gm. qd × 3 d. 11/15. *L. atkinson R.N.*
g. Correctly explaining how to cope with short-term illness and manage her diabetes.	g. Goal not met. Patient says she rarely is ill and doesn't feel diabetes will be affected. 11/15. *L. atkinson R.N.*
h. Purchasing medic alert tag.	h. Goal met. Medic alert tag for diabetes purchased through hospital. 11/13. *L. atkinson R.N.*
2. Fear of diabetic complications to be based on verbalization of accurate data regarding progress and complications of adult onset diabetes mellitus by 11/10.	2. Goal met. Patient discussed realistic diabetic complications and prevention. *11/10 L. atkinson R.N.*
3. Verbalizations of feelings related to diabetes indicating positive self-concept by 11/12.	3. Goal not met. Patient feels anger over diagnosed diabetic condition. Feels if she had controlled her weight better in the past she could have prevented it. 11/12. *L. atkinson R.N.*

The care plan for Mrs. Witten, developed in Chapters 1 and 2, follows with the addition of evaluation of goal achievement.

NURSING CARE PLAN FOR MRS. WITTEN

Goals

1. Patient to report pain management techniques adequate preoperatively

2. Patient to state feeling less fearful of hospital and illness prior to surgery

3. Patient will verbalize course of events for surgery and activities to prevent postop problems within 24h

4. Demonstrate breast self-exam before discharge

Evaluation of Goal Achievement

1. Goal met. Patient reported pain tolerable with analgesics
   6/4/86 L. Atkinson

2. Goal met. Patient still reported being "scared" of surgery several hours preop but not as "terrified" as when first admitted.
   6/4/86 Atkinson

3. Goal partially met. Patient described preop and surgical events but stated she "really did not care what happened to her after surgery as long as she made it through the surgery, the recovery would be easy."
   6/4/86 Atkinson

4. Goal met. Patient demonstrated breast self-exam correctly on morning of discharge.
   6/8/86 L. Atkinson

REVIEW OF THE NURSING PROCESS

Following evaluation of goal achievement, the nurse reviews the entire nursing process and the plan of care. This is done whether the goal was achieved or not. Review of the nursing process keeps the plan of nursing care current and responsive to the patient's changing needs. The process of nursing is not just sequential, consisting of steps 1 through 4 and then you are done. The process of nursing is cyclical in nature with the steps of assessment, planning, implementation, and evaluation viewed as a circle with one step leading to another. The nursing care a person receives reflects the changing health status of the patient, medical treatment changes, environmental changes, and the changing needs of the

patient and family. This is accomplished through the activities of nursing process review. This review process is spelled out in the *Standards of
Nursing Practice* (ANA, 1976):

> VIII. The client's/patient's progress or lack of progress toward goal
> achievement directs reassessment, reordering of priorities, new goal set-
> ting, and revision of the plan of nursing care.

$$\text{Review of the Nursing Process} = \text{Reassessment} + \text{Replanning} + \text{Review of Implementation}$$

Review of the nursing process consists of activities already described in the previous chapters: assessment (reassessment), planning
(replanning), implementation (review of implementation). This process
of review results in an updated plan for nursing care, which is then im-
plemented and evaluated, leading again to review as part of evaluation.
(See Figure 4–2.)

Reassessment

During the activity of reassessment, the nurse:

1. Examines old data to decide whether it still represents the patient accurately.
2. Examines new data gathered during interaction with the patient to determine whether new concerns or problems are
   present.
3. Examines previously written nursing diagnoses to determine
   whether they have been resolved or whether they remain current problems for the patient.
4. Identifies new nursing diagnoses based on data review.
5. Updates the care plan to reflect new and resolved diagnoses.

For example, during evaluation the patient demonstrated goal
achievement. During reassessment it was determined that the problem
identified in the diagnosis no longer existed. The nurse documents goal
achievement in the patient's chart and indicates that the diagnosis was
resolved on the care plan.

NURSING DIAGNOSIS: Potential impairment of skin integrity
    related to immobility.

LONG-TERM GOAL: Patient will maintain skin integrity during period of immobility.

EVALUATION: (To be done only after patient becomes mobile again, i.e., improved condition, changed medical orders.) Goal met; patient's skin integrity maintained while on bedrest. 11/13.

L. Atkinson R.N.

REASSESSMENT: Problem related to immobility no longer exists. Patient now ambulatory. 11/13: Care plan related to this problem is discontinued.

L. Atkinson R.N.

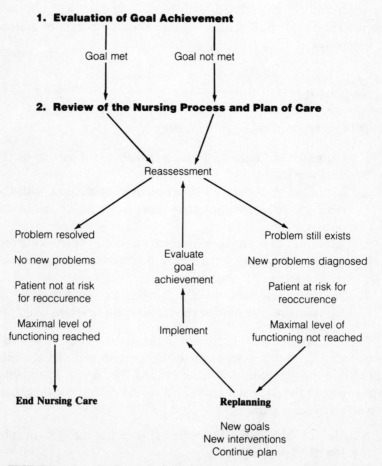

1. Evaluation of Goal Achievement

Goal met   Goal not met

2. Review of the Nursing Process and Plan of Care

Reassessment

Problem resolved   Problem still exists

No new problems   Evaluate   New problems diagnosed
                           goal
Patient not at risk   achievement   Patient at risk for
for reoccurence   reoccurence

Maximal level of   Implement   Maximal level of
functioning reached   functioning not reached

End Nursing Care   **Replanning**

                           New goals
                           New interventions
                           Continue plan

FIGURE 4–2.   Evaluation flow chart.

If the goal was not achieved, reassessment may help to point out reasons for this, such as inaccurate or incomplete data, inaccurate analysis of the data resulting in an invalid nursing diagnosis, or the development of new problems that interfered with the original plan. If the goal was met and the problem resolved, the nurse considers the need for preventive nursing care if the patient is still at risk.

Replanning

During the activity of replanning, the nurse

1. Reexamines priorities among the nursing diagnoses remaining on the patient's care plan to determine whether the ordering is still appropriate. Priorities are reordered as needed based on new data indicating more critical problems.
2. Examines previous goals to determine whether they are still valid or whether they should be changed to reflect a changed patient status.
3. Deletes goals associated with resolved diagnoses from the care plan. Deletes interventions associated with resolved diagnoses from the care plan.
4. Selects new goals for new diagnoses identified during reassessment.
5. Examines nursing interventions selected in the original plan to determine whether they should continue unchanged or whether a different approach would be more effective.

For example:

NURSING DIAGNOSIS: Alterations in nutrition: more than body requirements
NURSING GOALS:
Long-term: Weight of 130 lb by 9/30 (patient's goal)
Short-term:
Weight of 201 lb by 1/14.
Weight of 199 lb by 1/21.
Weight of 197 lb by 1/28.
(2 lb per week average weight loss)
EVALUATION:
Short-term goal—
Goal met. Weight of 201 lb 1/14.
Goal met. Weight of 199 lb 1/21

Goal met. Weight of 197 lb 1/28.

Goal met. Weight of 195 lb 2/4.

REASSESSMENT: *After short-term goal achieved*. Patient is los-
ing weight. Problem still exists. Continue diagnosis.

REPLANNING: Advance to next progressive short-term goal.
"Weight of 193 by 2/11." Continue current interventions.

REASSESSMENT: *After long-term goal achieved*. Patient has
reached end-goal weight.

Problem of "overweight" no longer exists.

New diagnosis: Alterations in nutrition: Potential for more than
   body requirements related to recent weight loss history.

REPLANNING:

New goal: Maintain current weight within 3 lb for 1 yr.

New nursing plan:

1. Weekly weigh-in 2 × mo, × 6 mo then q. mo × 6 mo.

2. Gradually add food to diet until intake 1200–1500 cal. per d.

3. Encourage *daily* weight monitoring at home with diet ad-
justed on daily basis to maintain weight.

4. Discuss continuing with exercise program of walking 2
miles q.d.

R
E
V
I
E
W

Review of Implementation. During review of the implementation
phase of the nursing process, the nurse examines what actually happened with the patient during nursing care. Factors such as the environment, the nurse's skills and knowledge, and the patient's responses are
considered. This is where the nurse evaluates personal behavior in rela-
tion to giving patient care. Does the nurse require further skills or information to be more effective? Did the nurse's personal feelings affect
the quality of care delivered to the patient? Were the interventions realistic in terms of time and resources? Were the interventions carried out
by other nursing personnel? If not, why not? Were the interventions too
vague or misinterpreted? Review of what occurred during implementation of the original nursing plan of care may point out problems that
can be corrected as the plan is updated. This is especially important
when the goal was not achieved. Evaluation, consisting of evaluation of
goal achievement and review of the nursing process and plan of care,
helps the nurse develop the skills of writing realistic and effective care
plans for dealing with patient's problems.

The care plan for Mrs. Witten follows with the addition of the second part of evaluation, review of the nursing process, and plan of care.
The completed abbreviated care plan follows nursing process review
and demonstrates how the care plan might look on a nursing Kardex.

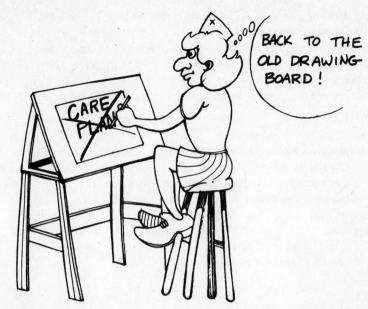

FIGURE 4–3. Review of the nursing process leads to revision of the existing care plan.

NURSING CARE PLAN FOR MRS. WITTEN

Review of the Nursing Process and Plan of Care

Reassessment:
data:

- transferred back to station after several hours in recovery following cholecystectomy
- IV infusing at 125 cc/hour per doctor's order
- Penrose drain in place draining blood-tinged bile
- ½-inch drainage area on incisional dressing
- nasogastric tube in place draining gastric contents on low suction per doctor's order for 24 hours
- NPO × 24 hours, then clear liquids to full as tolerated per doctor's order
- shallow respiration of 22–24 breaths/min
- patient reports incisional pain on movement/breathing in upper right quadrant of abdomen; requesting pain relief
- patient states, "I'm so glad its over and I'm O.K."

new diagnoses:

Alteration in comfort: incisional pain postcholecystectomy

Alterations in nutrition: less than body requirements related to NPO and decreased bowel activity

Potential impairment in skin integrity related to drainage from Penrose
    drain at incisional site
Ineffective breathing patterns related to incisional pain on inspiration
Probable knowledge deficit: inadequate information related to postop
    treatments and problem prevention
Resolution of previous problems associated with preoperative state

Replanning:
new goals:
1. Patient to report pain management techniques are adequate during
   postop period
2. Normal bowel sounds present by 24 hours postop
3. Maintenance of skin integrity at incisional site during postop period
4. Normal breath sounds and rate of 12–16 maintained during postop
   period
5. Patient to describe activities to prevent postop complications and
   normal course of recovery on first postop day

new plans:
for goal #1:
1. Assess for pain every 3–4 hours postop
2. Encourage the use of analgesics as ordered every 3 hours for moderate
   pain before it becomes severe
3. Assist with positioning every 2 hours
4. Assist to splint incision with blanket/pillow before coughing and deep
   breathing
5. Offer diversional activities: radio, TV
6. Offer backrub qhs—(at hour of sleep)

for goal #2:
1. Assess bowel sounds every 4 hours until active sounds heard
2. Maintain NPO status until bowel sounds present
3. Maintain IV infusion as ordered
4. Intake and output measurements × 48 hours
5. Encourage ambulation after operative day, 4 times a day, in halls
6. Reposition in bed every 2 hours day of surgery
7. Begin sips of clear liquids and advance to 500ml every 8 hours as tolerated

for goal #3:
1. Assess dressings every 2 hours; change PRN
2. Clean area under dressings every 8 hours with water; dry before re-
   placing dressings
3. Warm air to skin under dressings for 3 minutes every 4 hours on low
   setting if redness or skin irritation develops (use hair dryer)

for goal #4:
1. Assess breath sounds every 4 hours

2. Assist to take sustained maximal inspirations every hour; cough if
   secretions present (deep breath held for 3 seconds before expiration)
3. Low Fowler's position in bed; change position every 2 hours
4. Ambulate 4 times a day, in halls

for goal #5:

1. Assess knowledge after return from surgery
2. Describe medical orders related to tubes, diet, IV infusion, activity
   level, analgesics
3. Explain preventive care for skin and respiratory functioning

Plan Revised: 6/4/86 L. Atkinson R.N.

NURSING CARE PLAN FOR MRS. WITTEN

Nursing Diagnoses	Goals	Interventions	Evaluation
Alt. in comfort: acute pain r/t prob. gallbladder disease	Pt. states pain mgmt. adeq. preop	1. Assess for activ. that precip./intensify pain and avoid. Enc. activ. pt. uses to reduce pain if safe 2. Assess pain q3h; offer analg. q3h as ordered 3. Aqua-k heating pad to abdomen as pt. desires 4. Assist with positioning q2h	Goal met. Pt. reported pain tolerable with analgesics 6/4/86 L. Atkinson R.N.
Fear r/t uncertain outcome and hospitalization	Pt. state less fearful of hosp. and illness b/4 surgery	1. Pain management first 2. Assess understanding of dx/tx and give info prn 3. Orient to room, equip. and schedules for next 3–4h 4. Enc. husband to stay 5. Assign same nurses to care 6. Enc. verbalization of fears 7. Assess q1–2h; answer call light promptly	Goal met. Pt still reporting "scared" of surgery but not as "terrified" as on admission 6/4/86 L. Atkinson R.N.

| Know. deficit: insuf. know. r/t surgical tx | Pt. state events r/t surgery and activ. to prevent post-op prob. in next 24h | 1. Assess understanding of info. from M.D. and reinforce
2. Discuss preop, OR, and postop exp. with family
3. Discuss pain mgmt., common physical sensations
4. Give printed info, chole.
5. Return for quest. 2–3h b/4 surgery | Goal partially met. Pt. described preop and OR events but stated "did not care what happened to her after surgery—as long as she made it through, recovery would be easy." 9/4/86 L. Atkinson R.N. |
| Health maint. deficit: inability to do SBE r/t lack of information | Demo. SBE before discharge | 1. Explain impt. of early detec. and tx
2. Timing of SBE q month 1–2 days after menstru.
3. Demo. of exam for pt.
4. ID abnor. findings to report stat to MD
5. Give printed info on SBE
9/3/86 L. Atkinson R.N. | Goal met. Pt demo. SBE correctly 9/8/86 M. Murray R.N. |

BIBLIOGRAPHY

ANA: Standards for Nursing Practice. Kansas City, 1973. #NP.41.

Atkinson, L., and Murray, M. E.: Fundamentals of Nursing: A Nursing Process Approach. Macmillan, New York, 1985.

Campbell, C.: Nursing Diagnosis and Intervention in Nursing Practice, 2nd ed. Wiley, New York, 1984.

Carlson, J., Craft, C., and McGuire, A.: Nursing Diagnosis. Saunders, Philadelphia, 1982.

Carnevali, D.: Nursing Care Planning: Diagnosis and Management, 3rd ed. Lippincott, Philadelphia, 1983.

Carpenito, L. J.: Nursing Diagnosis Application to Clinical Practice. Lippincott, Philadelphia, 1983.

Doenges, M., Jeffries, M., and Moorhouse, M.: Nursing Care Plans: Nursing Diagnoses. In: Planning Patient Care. Davis, Philadelphia, 1984.

Gordon, M.: Nursing Diagnosis. McGraw-Hill, New York, 1982.

Griffith, J., and Christensen, P.: Nursing Process: Application of Theories, Frameworks, and Models. Mosby, St. Louis, 1982.

Hampshire, G.: Defining Goals. Nursing Times, March 16, 1983. 79(11): 45–46.

JCAH: Accreditation Manual for Hospitals. Chicago, 1985.

Kim, M., and Moritz, D.: Classification of Nursing Diagnoses: Proceedings of the Third and Fourth National Conferences. McGraw-Hill, New York, 1982.

Kim, M., McFarland, G., and McLane, A.: Classification of Nursing Diagnoses: Proceedings of the Fifth National Conference. Mosby, St. Louis, 1984.

LaMonica, E.: The Humanistic Nursing Process. Wadsworth, CA, 1985.

Lewis, S., and Collier, I.: Medical-Surgical Nursing: Assessment and Management of Clinical Problems. McGraw-Hill, New York, 1983.

Nursing: A Social Policy Statement. ANA, 1980. Publication #63-35M-12/80.

Olds, S., London, M., and Ladewig, P.: Maternal Newborn Nursing—A Family Centered Approach, 2nd ed. Addison-Wesley, Menlo Park, CA, 1984.

Sanborn, C., and Blount, M.: Standard Care Plans for Care and Discharge. Am. J. Nurs., Nov. 1984, 84(11):1394–96.

Yura, H., and Walsh, M.: The Nursing Process, 4th ed. Appleton-Century, Crofts, Norwalk, CT, 1983.

Sample Nursing Care Plans

1. **Infant:** Cleft Lip Repair
2. **Toddler:** Viral Croup
3. **School Age:** Seizure
4. **Adolescent:** Motorcycle Accident
5. **Early Adult:** Standardized Computerized Care Plan—Postpartum
6. **Middle Adult:** Heart Attack
7. **Senior Adult:** Depression

NURSING CARE PLAN #1
DATA COLLECTION AND ANALYSIS

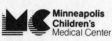
Minneapolis Children's Medical Center

2525 Chicago Avenue
Minneapolis, Minnesota 55404

Peterson, James
195638-3 R-243
1/5/86　2 weeks old

Race _Caucasian_ Height _22"_ Weight _8lb. 9oz_ T _98°_ ax P _120_ R _32_ BP _90/50_ OFC _14"_

Date _1/5/86_ Time of arrival _8 AM_ Person interviewed/Relationship _mother_ Phone _881-1257_

Language of parents _English_ of child _preverbal_ Interpreter name/phone _NA_

Person child lives with _mother + father_ Unusual circumstances influencing interview _NA_

Circumstances leading to this hospitalization? reason for bringing your child to the hospital? _repair of birth defect - cleft lip_

What has the doctor told you about your child's illness? tests, surgery, etc.? _3 days in hospital; mom can hold during induction of anesthesia_

Has the child been exposed to any communicable diseases?　Y　Ⓝ　what? _____ when? _____

Name of child's doctor _Johnson, David_ City/State _Mpls, Minnesota_

Name of child's dentist _Isaacson_ City/State _Mpls, Minnesota_

Any previous hospitalizations?　Y　Ⓝ　hospital _____ when? _____ why? _____

What was the child and parents' reaction to the hospitalization? _NA_

Has the child been receiving any medications at home?　Y　Ⓝ　any allergies?　Y　Ⓝ　reactions?　Y　N

medication	dose/frequency	last given	food allergy	drug allergy	type of reaction

NURSING HISTORY (0-5 YEARS)

Family/Home background	Habits of daily living - food/fluids	
• nickname _Jamie_	• likes _uses cleft lip nipple for fdg._	• bed climber?　Y　N　_NA_
• siblings (names/ages) _none_		• soother/special toy　_X_
	• dislikes	• special sleep habits　_X_
		Habits of daily living - elimination
	• type of formula _Similac c̄ Iron_	• usual bowel habits
• other important family members	• amount fdg. _2-3 oz_	• frequency _3-5 day_
June Peterson - mother	• frequency fdg. _2-5 l - demand_	• times
Robert " - father	• methods: cup bottle breast _NA_	
	• temp of fluids _room temp_	• terms for stool _NA_
• household pets	• type of solids: strain puree chop	• terms for urine _X_
	• frequency meals	• uses: potty toilet _X_
• lodging if out-of-town _NA_	• frequency snacks	• toilet trained?　Y　Ⓝ
• visiting plans _stay overnight_	**Habits of daily living - sleep**	• diapers at night?　Ⓨ　N
• ways parents would like to participate in care _hold and comfort - feed if possible_	• bedtime _11 PM last fdg_	• bladder expression/enema _NA_
	• naptime _sleeps 2-5 hrs c̄ 4 fdg_	
• religion _Lutheran_ baptized?　Ⓨ　N	• sleeps through night?　Y　Ⓝ	

64-70167
Rev. 2/85

NURSING HISTORY (0-5 YEARS)　　　　　　　_Continue on reverse side_

Courtesy Minneapolis Children's Medical Center.

INFANT: CLEFT LIP REPAIR

Recreation and Sociability		Recreation and Sociability	
• favorite toys/activities	NA	• capabilities of physically &/or mentally handicapped:	
		restrictions/limitations -	none
• play with others or alone?	NA		
• language skills (special words)	NA	special braces/glasses -	NA
		self-help -	
• special belongings - are they with child? Y N	NA		
		mobility -	none
• used to baby sitters? Y N	No	feeding -	cleft lip nipple for fdgs
• previous experience away from home - day care, visits, etc.			
none		speech -,	none

PROBLEM - ORIENTED

SUBJECTIVE

Questions and special concerns of child/parents? Do parents understand orientation to child's room, nursing unit, isolation rooms?

Mother: "I'll be so glad when this is over. My poor baby. Is this going to hurt him? I want to be with him as much as possible. Will they put needles or tubes in him?"

Father: asking about staying overnight with baby.

OBJECTIVE

Observations made during interview? parents' reactions? parent-child interaction? Mother tearful; holding baby close; baby alert, quiet in mothers arms demonstrated use of nurse call, light and crib rails
- cleft on left side of mouth, ½ way up to nose; palate intact
- baby has regained birthweight + 5 oz.

ASSESSMENT

Nursing assessment of child on admission? physical appearance? adjustment to hospital? Neonate in stable condition on admission to hospital. 1/5/86 for repair of cleft lip at 10³⁰ AM today. Basic needs met adequately by parents. Alert and quiet with mother holding. Parents knowledge of preop-OK-post op course limited to use of general anesthesia and repair of lip

PLAN

Problems identified for patient care plan Diagnoses:	Goals
1. Anxiety of parents related to surgery and hospitalization	1. Parents to state less anxious by 10 AM 1/6
2. Potential alteration in comfort: pain following cleft lip repair	2. Little or no crying post-op
3. Knowledge deficit: parents not familiar with medical + nsg tx pre-post op	3. Parents to discuss pre post op tx for baby by 10 AM 1/6
4. Potential feeding problems post-op related to discomfort	4. Oral intake of 12 oz / day 1/6, 7, 8

Signature/Title Leslie Atkinson R.N.   Date 1/5/86   Time 8 15 AM

NURSING HISTORY (0-5 YEARS)

NURSING CARE PLAN #1 (Cont.)

Planned Actions	*Rationale*
1. a. Reassure parents regarding surgery and postop course.	**1. a.** Information about surgery and tx often decreases anxiety of unknown.
b. Enc. parents' involvement in tx and prep for surgery.	**b.** Maintaining parental roles decreases stress for family.
c. Take parents to waiting room after anesth. induct. and assure them of M.D. visit immed. postop.	**c.** Physical comfort of parents; immediate info from M.D. postop for actual outcome reduces stress.
d. Offer hosp. facilities: cafeterial, chapel, lounge.	**d.** Comfort of religious beliefs; meeting parents' physical needs.
2. a. Talk with parents about role in holding/touching infant to keep him calm.	**2. a.d.** Crying causes tension on suture line. Facilitate parent/infant bonding.
b. Maintain warmth.	**b.c.d.** Infants' needs for warmth, food, and love are communicated through crying when needs are unmet.
c. Maintain demand feeding pattern.	
d. Pick up infant and cuddle/rock when crying first begins.	
3. a. Provide time for family to adjust to hospital b/4 providing information.	**3. a.** Familiarity with environment decreases stress and promotes learning.
b. Two hours preop provide printed info. on cleft lip repair.	**b.** Printed info. allows parents to learn at own pace and reinforces teaching of M.D. and nurse.
c. Discuss info. on pre-postop tx for baby and parents' questions 1 hour preop.	**c.** Increases learning and decreases stress related to unknown.
d. Explain all tx to parents b/4 implementing.	**d.** Knowledge of tx decreases parents' anxiety.
4. a. Hold infant upright for all feedings.	**4. a.** Gravity assists formula into stomach.
b. Feed slowly with Asepto syringe $\bar{c}$ 1½" rubber catheter extension, 3–4 oz q3–4 h.	**b.** Unfamiliar feeding method for infant. Sucking prohibited due to stress it would put on sutures.
c. Frequent bubbling.	**c.** Increased swallowing of air with Asepto.

INFANT: CLEFT LIP REPAIR

Planned Actions

    d. Catheter placed inside of mouth and formula put on top of tongue.

    e. Hold for 10–15 min following feeding. Encourage parent to hold.

    f. Lay on side following feeding.

    g. Feed infant on a demand schedule.

    1/5/86 L. Atkinson R.N.

Rationale

    d. Prevent attempt at sucking and facilitate swallowing.

    e. Safety/security need; calm infant less likely to regurgitate or aspirate feeding.

    f. If emesis occurs, side position facilitates drainage.

    g. Helps prevent aspiration. Infant crying causes trauma to suture line. Hunger increases ease of feeding.

NURSING CARE PLAN #1 (Cont.)

Evaluation

1. Goal met. Parents "doing much better" ½ hour preop.

   1/5/86 L. Atkinson R.N.

2. Goal not met. Jamie crying freq. during night.

   1/6/86 J. Lindstrom R.N.

3. Goal met. Parents stated understanding of pre- and postop tx for baby.

   1/5/86 L. Atkinson R.N.

4. Goal met. Intake of 12–16 oz each postop day.

   1/8/86 M. Thompson R.N.

Review of Nursing Process/ Care Plan

1. Problem still exists. New goal: Parents to report minimum anxiety 3–4h postop. Continue to reassure and inform.

2. Continue goal and actions. Enc. parents to hold baby during tx. of suture line on lip.

3. Problem still exists. New goal: Parents to state understanding of postop tx. Continue with interventions.

4. Able to take nipple feedings; discharge 1/8. Problem resolved.

NURSING CARE PLAN #2
DATA COLLECTION AND ANALYSIS

MC Minneapolis Children's Medical Center

2525 Chicago Avenue
Minneapolis, Minnesota 55404

Race _Caucasian_ Height _32"_ Weight _26 lbs_ T _102 (R)_ P _120_ R _40_ BP _100/70_ OFC _19"_

Date _2/14/86_ Time of arrival _6 PM_ Person interviewed/Relationship _Father_ Phone _325-1974_

Language of parents _English_ of child _English_ Interpreter name/phone_____

Person child lives with _parents_ Unusual circumstances influencing interview _admitted to ICU_

Circumstances leading to this hospitalization? reason for bringing your child to the hospital? _Croup; gasping for air at home; doctor told father to bring to emergency room._

What has the doctor told you about your child's illness? tests, surgery, etc.? _Croup; "bad narrowing of trachea"; doctor wants child in croup tent with oxygen_

Has the child been exposed to any communicable diseases? Y N what?_____ when?_____

Name of child's doctor _J. Larson_ City/State _Bloomington, Minnesota_

Name of child's dentist _Farber_ City/State _Bloomington, Minnesota_

Any previous hospitalizations? Y (N) hospital_____ when?_____ why?_____

What was the child and parents' reaction to the hospitalization?_____

Has the child been receiving any medications at home? Y (N) any allergies? Y (N) reactions? Y N

medication	dose/frequency	last given	food allergy	drug allergy	type of reaction

Family/Home background

- nickname _no_
- siblings (names/ages)
  Derik   5 yrs
- other important family members
  Ann James (mother)
  Steve James (father)
- household pets _cat & dog_
- lodging if out-of-town _NA_
- visiting plans _continuous_
- ways parents would like to participate in care _anyway they can_
- religion _Cath._ baptized? (Y) N

Habits of daily living · food/fluids

- likes _finger foods; feeds self; grape juice_
- dislikes _squash; tomatoes_
- type of formula _2% milk_
- amount fdg.
- frequency fdg. _3 meals + bedtime_
- methods: (cup) (bottle) breast _bottle_
- temp of fluids _cold_
- type of solids: strain puree (chop)
- frequency meals _3 x day_
- frequency snacks _in between x 2_

Habits of daily living - sleep

- bedtime _7 PM_
- naptime _1 - 2³⁰ p_
- sleeps through night? (Y) N

Habits of daily living

- bed climber? Y (N)
- soother/special toy _blanket_
- special sleep habits _story, bottle first, night light_

Habits of daily living - elimination

- usual bowel habits
- frequency _q day_
- times _am_
- terms for stool _poop_
- terms for urine _pee_
- uses: potty toilet _diapers_
- toilet trained? Y (N)
- diapers at night? (Y) N
- bladder expression/enema _no_

NURSING HISTORY (0-5 YEARS)

64-70167
Rev. 2/85

NURSING HISTORY (0-5 YEARS)   Continue on reverse side

Courtesy Minneapolis Children's Medical Center.

TODDLER: VIRAL CROUP

Recreation and Sociability	Recreation and Sociability
• favorite toys/activities _tractors, "Sesame Street"_	• capabilities of physically &/or mentally handicapped:
	restrictions/limitations - _none._
• play with others or alone? _alone_	
• language skills (special words) _mama, dada, no, hot_	special braces/glasses · _NA_
	self-help · _help c̄ all needs_
• special belongings - are they with child? (Y) N _blanket_	
	mobility - _walks, runs, climbs_
• used to baby sitters? Y N _once a month_	feeding - _self, holds own bottle_
• previous experience away from home - day care, visits, etc. _none_	_minimal spilling with cup_
	speech _understands most of what is said according to father_

PROBLEM - ORIENTED

SUBJECTIVE

Questions and special concerns of child/parents? Do parents understand orientation to child's room, nursing unit, isolation rooms? "_He collapsed at home, gasping for air. I didn't know what to do but I knew he was bad. The doctor saw him in the emergency room and said David was going to the critical area. He needs oxygen and some moisture. We were using the shower and vaporizer at home, but it wasn't enough._"

OBJECTIVE

Observations made during interview? parents' reactions? parent-child interaction? _Inspiratory stridor with each breath; crying off and on; mother was notified at school of David's admission; suprasternal retractions and nasal flaring; alert; PCO_2 = 48 mm Hg (normal 35-45); crying during procedures; put in croup tent c̄ 30% O_2; NPO; IV started - D_5W at 40 cc/hr; holds tightly to blanket_

ASSESSMENT

Nursing assessment of child on admission? physical appearance? adjustment to hospital? _18 mo. old male child admitted to ICU via ER for severe respiratory distress from croup. Father comforting child but continues to cry freq. Pale, alert, working hard to breathe._

PLAN

Problems identified for patient care plan _Nursing Diagnoses:_

1. _Ineffective airway clearance related narrowed trachea from croup._
2. _Fear related to hospitalization and breathing difficulty_

Goals:
1. _Next blood gases in 2h show PCO_2 below 48 mm Hg_
2. _No crying during next 4h unless physically hurt_

Signature/Title _L. Adams R.N._ Date _2/14/86_ Time _6 ³⁰ P_

NURSING HISTORY (0-5 YEARS)

NURSING CARE PLAN #2 (Cont.)

Planned Actions	*Rationale*
1. **a.** Maintain O_2 at 40%.	1. **a.** Medical order.
b. Check O_2 concentration every ½h. while in croup tent.	**b.** Keep at ordered concentration.
c. Elevate head of bed 30°–60°.	**c.** Assist respirations—better lung expansion.
d. Encourage parent(s) to sit by bed or get under croup tent to hold/touch baby.	**d.g.h.** Familiar people/things will decrease stress of strange environment. Stress can contribute to respiratory distress.
e. Ensure adequate warmth/do not overheat.	**e.** Cold or heat stress increase metabolic O_2 requirements.
f. Disturb baby as little as possible.	**f.** Respiratory rate increases with excitement and/or fear.
g. Keep blanket within his reach.	
h. Keep parent(s) with baby during procedures.	
2. **a.** Talk to parents about role in calming baby; stay where baby can see them, touch/hold baby inside croup tent, stay with baby during night.	2. **a.b.c.** Familiar people/things will decrease stress of strange environment and provide psychological security.
b. Keep blanket with him at all times.	
c. Have parent(s) assist with procedures.	
d. Explain procedures and equipment to baby in simple terms. Let baby touch equipment before procedure, if possible.	**d.** Minimize fear of unknown.

Plan developed: 2/4/86 L. Adams RN.

TODDLER: VIRAL CROUP

Evaluation

1. Goal met; $PCO_2 = 46$ mm Hg. after 2h.

    2/14 10 P.M. *L. Adams RN.*

2. Goal met; baby cried only during venipuncture during last 4h.

    2/15 12 MN *K. Baker R.N.*

Review of Nursing Process/Care Plan

1. Continue goal and nursing actions and reevaluate in 2 more h after next blood gas results.

2. Continue goal and nursing actions and reevaluate in 4h.
    New Goal: Baby will sleep at least 6h during the 11 P.M.–7 A.M. shift.
    Planned Actions: Same as for Goal 2, but add "darken room."

NURSING CARE PLAN #3
DATA COLLECTION AND ANALYSIS

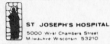

ST JOSEPH'S HOSPITAL
5000 West Chambers Street
Milwaukee Wisconsin 53210

NURSING
HISTORY &
ASSESSMENT

Jessica E. Knedle
Age 7 yrs.- Dr. A. Teston
3445925

PART A   (MEDICAL · SURGICAL)

DATE OF HISTORY	TIME OF HISTORY	INFORMANT(S)
11-22-86	7³⁰ a.m.	Mother of patient: Mrs. Mary Knedle

ADMITTING MEDICAL DIAGNOSIS
Grand mal seizure

ARRIVED ON UNIT: ☐ AMBULATORY ☐ WHEELCHAIR ☐ CART ☒ AMBULANCE

REASONS FOR HOSPITALIZATION
Pt. suffered seizure at home which mother (a nurse)
describes as grand mal & lasting 2 minutes

HOW HAS THE PATIENT BEEN MANAGING THE ABOVE PROBLEMS AT HOME?
First time this has happened

OTHER ILLNESSES OR CONDITIONS (HYPERTENSION, ARTHRITIS, DIABETES, PAST SURGERIES, ETC.)	ALLERGIES (FOOD, MEDICATION, TAPE, DYE, ETC.)
Child carries diagnosis of cerebral palsy - only apparent sign is Ⓛ foot turning inward.	none

ALCOHOL USAGE	LAST PHYSICIAL EXAM	TYPE OF REACTION
NA	1 year	none

MEDICATION AND DOSAGE PRESCRIBED AND NON-PRESCRIBED	USUAL TIMES TAKEN	TIME OF LAST DOSE	PATIENT'S UNDERSTANDING OF PURPOSE
none			

SUBJECTIVE DATA	OBJECTIVE DATA

COGNITION SENSATION/COMMUNICATION

LIMITATIONS OR RESTRICTIONS RELATED TO:
VISION: ☒ YES ☐ NO   HEARING: ☐ YES ☐ NO   OTHER: ☐ YES ☐ NO
DESCRIBE:
child states: "I'm so sleepy. Where am
I? Stay with me Mother".

LAST EYE EXAM
1 year

LEVEL OF ORIENTATION (ALERTNESS, ABILITY TO PROCESS INFORMATION, ETC.)
Not responsive in ER - groggy &
sleepy @ present.

GLASSES yes
CONTACT LENSES
ARTIFICIAL EYE
HEARING AID

APPEARANCE OF EYES, EARS, SPEECH IMPAIRMENTS, ETC.
No speech at present
Eyes closed

VENTILATION

REPORT OF DYSPNEA, COUGH, ORTHOPNEA, ETC "breathing funny"
Mo. states child was   just before seizure -
HOW MUCH DOES
PATIENT SMOKE? N.A. "fast & loud"

BREATH SOUNDS, SPUTUM, ETC.
Lungs clear

| RESP. RATE | 22 | DEPTH & QUALITY | Shallow |

© ST. JOSEPH'S HOSPITAL, MILWAUKEE, WISCONSIN 1982

SIGNATURE _____ P. Leiff R.N.

FORM 20441 REV. 5/84

NURSING HISTORY & ASSESSMENT · PART A

Courtesy St. Joseph's Hospital, Milwaukee, Wisconsin.

SCHOOL AGE: SEIZURE

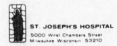

ST. JOSEPH'S HOSPITAL
5000 West Chambers Street
Milwaukee Wisconsin 53210

NURSING HISTORY & ASSESSMENT

(MEDICAL-SURGICAL)

PART B

SUBJECTIVE DATA	OBJECTIVE DATA
CIRCULATION REPORT OF CHEST PAIN, NUMBNESS, TINGLING, ETC. Child unresponsive verbally. while in ER no pain	PERIPHERAL PULSES, CAPILLARY REFILL, HOMAN'S SIGN, EDEMA, ETC. Pulse full, capillary refill brisk TEMP **98** ☐ O ☐ AX ☒ R PULSES☐ AP ☒ R **90** QUALITY ____ BP **110/60** ☐ R ☐ L ☒ LYING ☐ SITTING ☐ STANDING
NUTRITION/HYDRATION REPORTS OF ANOREXIA, NAUSEA, USUAL MEAL PATTERN, ABILITY TO CHEW AND SWALLOW, RECENT CHANGE IN WEIGHT, ETC. "Not fussy eater" "c̄ nausea @ 4 am" THERAPEUTIC DIET none LAST DENTAL EXAM 6 mo. ago	SKIN TURGOR, APPEARANCE OF TONGUE, CONDITION OF TEETH, ETC. mucous membranes intact HEIGHT WEIGHT DENTURES none
ELIMINATION BOWEL HABITS, VOIDING PATTERN, HEMORRHOIDS, DESCRIPTION OF MENSTRUAL CYCLE, ETC. mo. reports soiled self (urine) p̄ seizure REPORTED LBM 11-21 LAST PAP SMEAR LAST PROCTOSCOPIC EXAM	DIAPHORESIS, BOWEL SOUNDS, APPEARANCE OF URINE, FECES, VOMITUS, ETC. No emesis
MOBILITY REPORTED INABILITY TO DO ADLS, DIFFICULTY WITH AMBULATION, ETC. Mother reports child can swim, bike, roller skate". No problems from CP."	ROM, GAIT, STRENGTH, ENDURANCE, ETC. Not responding to commands at present CANE ____ CRUTCHES ____ WALKER ____ PROSTHESIS ____
INTEGUMENTARY REPORTED PRURITIS, ECZEMA, PSORIASIS, ETC. none LAST SELF-BREAST EXAM NA	INSPECTION FOR RASHES, OPEN AREAS, AND ABNORMAL NAIL CONDITION, ETC. NOTE DISTRIBUTION AND QUALITY OF HAIR OR PRESENCE OF WIG none ; pale skin, warm, moist
COMFORT SLEEP - REST REPORT OF PAIN, QUALITY, LOCATION, PRECIPITATING FACTORS, DURATION AND HOW PAIN IS RELIEVED none REPORTED SLEEP PATTERNS AND BEDTIME RITUALS 8 PM bedtime - sleeps 7-8 am	FACIAL GRIMACING, GUARDING OF AFFECTED AREA, ETC. (NOTE: THERE MAY BE NO OBSERVABLE SIGNS WITH CHRONIC PAIN.) Slight muscle twitching Ⓛ hand while in ER -
PSYCHOSOCIAL DESCRIBE MEMBERS OF SUPPORT SYSTEM OR IMMEDIATE HOUSEHOLD (AGE, HEALTH STATUS, ETC.) PATIENT'S RESPONSE TO CHANGE OR STRESS.	OBSERVED NON-VERBAL BEHAVIOR, INTERACTIONS WITH SIGNIFICANT OTHERS, ETC. Mother crying & states, "I'm so scared. She's such a bright child. Will she be OK? This has never happened before... aren't all these drugs bad for her?"

OCCUPATION AND/OR INTERESTS
Reads, draws, active child normally

DESCRIPTION OF HOME ENVIRONMENT
Lives in single family home with 2 brothers (10,8) and sister (8), father

UTILIZATION OF COMMUNITY RESOURCES	TYPE OF SERVICE PROVIDED
☐ VNA ☐ PHN ☐ OTHER: none	none

© ST. JOSEPH'S HOSPITAL - MILWAUKEE, WISCONSIN 1982

FORM 20523 1/82

SIGNATURE _____ P. Lieff _____ RN

NURSING HISTORY & ASSESSMENT - PART B

NURSING CARE PLAN #3 (Cont.)

Nursing Diagnosis

1. Potential for injury related to seizures.

2. Fear related to uncertain outcome. (This diagnosis pertains to the mother.)

Goals

1. Patient will suffer no physical injury related to seizures during hospitalization.

2. Mother will state accurate description of child's condition and prognosis by 4 P.M. 11/22.

Planned Actions

1. a. Continuous observation of child.
   b. Padded side rails up at all times.
   c. Padded tongue blade and airway at bedside.
   d. Vital signs and neuro checks q15 min × 8, q½ h × 8, q1h × 4.

   e. Orient mother/child.

2. a. Clarify and repeat info given by physicians to mother.

   b. Assess mother's understanding of info.
   c. Correct any misunderstanding and repeat correct info.

   d. Assist mother in explaining info to husband when he arrives.
   e. Explain all procedures done for child.
   f. Provide data from vital signs and neurochecks for parents.

   g. Provide and encourage rest opportunities for parents.

Rationale

1. a. Physical safety need.

   b.c. Protection should another or repeated seizures occur.

   d. Physical safety. Assessment of motor function and verbal responses provides diagnostic data.
   e. Psychological safety. Provide comfortable, secure environment.

2. a. A person experiencing stress may not accurately comprehend information given.
   b. Increase database for further nursing intervention.
   c. Simple, correct explanations, repeated frequently, are more likely to be understood during stress.
   d. Ensure accuracy of info given to father.

   e.f. The frequency of checks and procedures may cause parents unnecessary fear. Understanding procedures may reduce fear.
   g. Stress consumes high amounts of physical energy.

SCHOOL AGE: SEIZURE

Evaluation

1. Goal met. No physical injury. No recurrent seizures.
   11/24 _P. Reiff RN._
2. Goal met. Mother states: "This seizure was related to her CP and we can control it with medication, which she may be on for some years."
   11/22 _P. Reiff RN_

Review of Nursing Process/ Care Plan
New Nursing Diagnoses

3. Knowledge deficit related to care of child with seizure disorder.

4. Potential for injury related to possible recurrence of seizures postdischarge.

5. Social isolation related to hospitalization.

Review of Nursing Process/ Care Plan
New Data:

1. Transfer to Pediatric Unit. 11/24.
2. Maintenance antiepileptic drug: Phenobarbital 30 mg. qd A.M. 40 mg. qd hs.
3. Child states, "I want to go home. There's nothing to do here. Mom, will you stay with me?"
4. Mother states, "How do I take care of her? What if this happens again, or at school? What about sports . . . she's so active."

New Goals

3. Mother will demonstrate an understanding of child's care related to diagnosis as evidenced by ability to (at time of discharge):
   —correctly administer antiepileptic drug.
   —describe side effects of drug.
   —describe dietary restrictions related to drug.
   —describe home care during seizure, minor illnesses, and use of nonprescription medications.
4. Patient and family will take following safety precautions:
   b. Inform school of diagnosis and emergency actions in event of seizure.
   b. Wear medic alert necklace/ bracelet.
   c. Identify activities requiring adult supervision.
5. Patient will play with another child 2h by 11/24—4 P.M.

NURSING CARE PLAN #4
DATA COLLECTION AND ANALYSIS

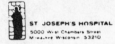

ST JOSEPH'S HOSPITAL
5000 West Chambers Street
Milwaukee Wisconsin 53210

NURSING HISTORY & ASSESSMENT

Jonathan C. Wilmont
Age 17 - 3619 Delaware S
5736-5768-75
Dr. R. Killan

PART A   (MEDICAL · SURGICAL)

DATE OF HISTORY	TIME OF HISTORY	INFORMANT(S)
11-15-86	6 PM.	Patient & parents

ADMITTING MEDICAL DIAGNOSIS | ARRIVED ON UNIT From E.R.
Neurologic Observation / Head Lacerations
☐ AMBULATORY   ___ WHEELCHAIR   ☒ CART   ☐ AMBULANCE

REASONS FOR HOSPITALIZATION
Driving motorcycle which skidded and overturned. Female passenger treated & released. Surgical cleansing of gravel under anesthesia.

HOW HAS THE PATIENT BEEN MANAGING THE ABOVE PROBLEMS AT HOME?

OTHER ILLNESSES OR CONDITIONS (HYPERTENSION, ARTHRITIS, DIABETES, PAST SURGERIES, ETC.)	ALLERGIES (FOOD, MEDICATION, TAPE, DYE, ETC.)
none	none

ALCOHOL USAGE	LAST PHYSICIAL EXAM	TYPE OF REACTION
"a beer now & then"	1985	

MEDICATION AND DOSAGE PRESCRIBED AND NON-PRESCRIBED	USUAL TIMES TAKEN	TIME OF LAST DOSE	PATIENT'S UNDERSTANDING OF PURPOSE

SUBJECTIVE DATA	OBJECTIVE DATA

COGNITION SENSATION/ COMMUNICATION

LIMITATIONS OR RESTRICTIONS RELATED TO:
VISION: ☐ YES ☒ NO   HEARING: ☐ YES ☒ NO   OTHER: ☐ YES ☒ NO
DESCRIBE:
Shouting "I'm not hurt bad. Why do I have to stay here c̄ you all poking at me."

LAST EYE EXAM   1985

LEVEL OF ORIENTATION (ALERTNESS, ABILITY TO PROCESS INFORMATION, ETC.)
Oriented to time, date, place

GLASSES ___ no
CONTACT LENSES ___
ARTIFICIAL EYE ___
HEARING AID ___

APPEARANCE OF EYES, EARS, SPEECH IMPAIRMENTS, ETC.
Pupils equal & reactive to light

VENTILATION

REPORT OF DYSPNEA, COUGH, ORTHOPNEA, ETC
"Of course I don't smoke."
HOW MUCH DOES PATIENT SMOKE?   none

BREATH SOUNDS, SPUTUM, ETC.
Lungs clear
RESP. RATE 26   DEPTH & QUALITY normal - effortless

ST. JOSEPH'S HOSPITAL, MILWAUKEE, WISCONSIN 1982

SIGNATURE _____ P. Burke _____ R.N

FORM 20441 REV. 5/84

NURSING HISTORY & ASSESSMENT - PART A

Courtesy St. Joseph's Hospital, Milwaukee, Wisconsin.

**ADOLESCENT:
MOTORCYCLE ACCIDENT**

NURSING
HISTORY &
ASSESSMENT

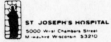

ST JOSEPH'S HOSPITAL
5000 West Chambers Street
Milwaukee Wisconsin 53210

(MEDICAL · SURGICAL)

PART B

SUBJECTIVE DATA	OBJECTIVE DATA
CIRCULATION REPORT OF CHEST PAIN, NUMBNESS, TINGLING, ETC. *No chest pain – Shouts "No, I won't wiggle my toes one more time."*	PERIPHERAL PULSES, CAPILLARY REFILL, HOMAN'S SIGN, EDEMA, ETC. *Pulses strong, refill brisk, neg Homan's* TEMP *99⁸* ☒O ☐AX ☐R PULSES☐AP ☒R *26* QUALITY ___ BP *110/76* ☐R ☒L ☒LYING ☐SITTING ☐STANDING
NUTRITION/ HYDRATION REPORTS OF ANOREXIA, NAUSEA, USUAL MEAL PATTERN, ABILITY TO CHEW AND SWALLOW, RECENT CHANGE IN WEIGHT, ETC. *"I'm hungry – can't you get me some decent food?."* THERAPEUTIC DIET *NPO × 24 hrs.* LAST DENTAL EXAM *'86*	SKIN TURGOR, APPEARANCE OF TONGUE, CONDITION OF TEETH, ETC. *Skin warm, dry* HEIGHT *5' 11"* WEIGHT *155* DENTURES *no*
ELIMINATION BOWEL HABITS, VOIDING PATTERN, HEMORRHOIDS, DESCRIPTION OF MENSTRUAL CYCLE, ETC. *daily BM "I'm getting up – I can't go in that" (urinal)* REPORTED LBM *11-14* LAST PAP SMEAR LAST PROCTOSCOPIC EXAM	DIAPHORESIS, BOWEL SOUNDS, APPEARANCE OF URINE, FECES, VOMITUS, ETC. *Lt. amber urine* *No diaphoresis*
MOBILITY REPORTED INABILITY TO DO ADLS, DIFFICULTY WITH AMBULATION, ETC. *"What do you mean bed rest – I'm not going to rot in here."*	ROM, GAIT, STRENGTH, ENDURANCE, ETC. *Strict bed rest ordered. Moves all extremities; grasp equal* CANE _____ CRUTCHES _____ WALKER _____ PROSTHESIS _____
INTEGUMENTARY REPORTED PRURITIS, ECZEMA, PSORIASIS, ETC. *"My head – I look awful."* LAST SELF BREAST EXAM	INSPECTION FOR RASHES, OPEN AREAS, AND ABNORMAL NAIL CONDITION, ETC. NOTE DISTRIBUTION AND QUALITY OF HAIR OR PRESENCE OF WIG *Dressings on arms/legs. (R) temporal area shaved - 12 stitches*
COMFORT SLEEP - REST REPORT OF PAIN, QUALITY, LOCATION, PRECIPITATING FACTORS, DURATION AND HOW PAIN IS RELIEVED *"My head feels bad – like a headache"* REPORTED SLEEP PATTERNS AND BEDTIME RITUALS *Bed @ 11PM Up by 7 am for school*	FACIAL GRIMACING, GUARDING OF AFFECTED AREA, ETC. (NOTE: THERE MAY BE NO OBSERVABLE SIGNS WITH CHRONIC PAIN.) *No complaints of pain other than head*
PSYCHOSOCIAL DESCRIBE MEMBERS OF SUPPORT SYSTEM OR IMMEDIATE HOUSEHOLD (AGE, HEALTH STATUS, ETC.) PATIENT'S RESPONSE TO CHANGE OR STRESS. *"Some mess I've made. My bike... what will Julie's (passenger) parents think? I wanted them to trust me."*	OBSERVED NON-VERBAL BEHAVIOR, INTERACTIONS WITH SIGNIFICANT OTHERS, ETC. *Mother holding son's hand, brushing hair – teary & weepy. Father present – states "It was an accident, no one is blaming you."*

OCCUPATION AND/OR INTERESTS *Sports (all!) Honor roll student*
DESCRIPTION OF HOME ENVIRONMENT *Lives c̄ parents & siblings (ages 10, 15) at home.*
Parents state, "We should never have given him that bike."

UTILIZATION OF COMMUNITY RESOURCES	TYPE OF SERVICE PROVIDED
☐VNA ☐PHN ☐OTHER: *none*	*none*

© ST. JOSEPH'S HOSPITAL - MILWAUKEE, WISCONSIN 1982

SIGNATURE ___*S. Burke*___

FORM 20523 1/82

NURSING HISTORY & ASSESSMENT - PART B

NURSING CARE PLAN #4 (Cont.)

Nursing Diagnoses

1. Ineffective individual coping related to hospitalization as evidenced by anger, shouting.
2. Disturbance in self-esteem related to accident and hospitalization.

Goals

1. Patient will verbalize anger and begin to explore reasons 11/16.
2. Patient will make two statements of positive self-regard within 48h 11/17.

Planned Actions

1. **a.** Approach: nonjudgmental.
   b. Reflect feeling statements to patient, to parents.
   c. Maintain eye contact with patient.
   d. Stay with patient, esp. after verbal outbursts.
   e. Acknowledge appropriateness of anger.
   f. Use open-ended questions to help identify reasons for anger.
   g. Explain nec. of procedures.

   h. Maximize privacy during care.
2. **a.** Explain procedures before beginning care.
   b. Maximize choices patient can make.

   c. Help patient to maintain grooming and wear own pajamas.

   d. Spend time with patient when no physical care is necessary.
   f. Provide privacy during phone calls and visiting hours.

Rationale

1. **a.b.** Encourages verbalization of concerns.

   c. Shows acceptance and respect.
   d. Shows acceptance of anger as legitimate feeling.
   e. Encourages therapeutic ventilation of feelings.
   f. Encourages patient to direct the communication.
   g. Patient more likely to cooperate if understands reason for care.
   h. Emphasis on sexual identity during adolescence.
2. **a.** Knowledge may decrease anxiety.
   b. Adolescent seeks decision making and control of environment.
   c. Adolescent developmental task is self-identity. Body image of increased importance to adolescent.
   d.e. Provide data for positive self-esteem.
   f. Maintain contact and identity with peer group.

ADOLESCENT: MOTORCYCLE ACCIDENT

Review of Nursing Process/
Care Plan

Evaluation

1. Goal met. "You're darn right I'm angry. I've really made a mess of a relationship with a person I really care about.
   11/16 *P. Burke R.N.*

2. Goal not met. Patient beginning to express guilt over pain he had caused his passenger and states, "How can I ever face her again?"
   11/17 *P. Burke RN.*

2. Continue goal and actions.
   New action: Assist patient to validate his current perceptions of relationship with his passenger, her parents, and his parents.

NURSING CARE PLAN #5

EARLY ADULT: STANDARD COMPUTERIZED CARE PLAN—POSTPARTUM

Nursing Diagnoses

Alteration in comfort:

Pain _____

_____

Alteration in elimination:

_____

_____

_____

Breastfeeding problems related to: _____

_____

_____

Supporting Data

Subjective data about discomfort from episiotomy, c-section incision, hemorrhoids, afterbirth contractions, breasts/nipples; bruising, swelling at site.

Urinary: decreased sensation of full bladder, inability to void, distended bladder, voiding in small amounts, Foley catheter, swelling around urinary meatus, laceration of urethral area.

Bowel: absence/reduced bowel sounds, general anesthesia, decreased activity post-c-section, NPO/clear liquids, laceration into rectum at delivery, fear of painful defecation, inability to defecate for several days, retained flatus/abdominal distention.

Newborn: sleepy, premature, weak suck, poor rooting reflex, small mouth.

Mother: flat/inverted nipples, fatigue, pain, awkward positioning, large nipples.

Potential for infection related to: _____

Parental knowledge/skill deficit related to: _____
_____
_____

Alterations in uterine involution related to: _____
_____

Episiotomy, lacerations, c-section, cracked nipples, blocked milk ducts, Foley catheter, delivery.

Newborn: parents state or demonstrate inability to diaper, feed, bathe, handle, transport in car, take temperature. Mother: unfamiliar with growth and development, contraception, self-care postpartum.

Excess vaginal bleeding, passing clots, soft uterus, uterus displaced to right or left above umbilicus, distended bladder, elevated pulse, low BP.

To the reader: This type of care plan would be printed by the computer printer following the command for a standard postpartum care plan with no identified complications. The nurse would then indicate on the printed plan the diagnoses and interventions most appropriate for this patient. The nurse would complete the diagnoses with the specific problem and etiology of the problem, if known, for this patient. Nursing interventions would be individualized by adding information and additional interventions not on the form. The nurse would also complete the evaluation of the plan for the individual patient.

EARLY ADULT: STANDARD COMPUTERIZED CARE PLAN— POSTPARTUM

NURSING CARE PLAN #5 (Cont.)

Goals of Care	Planned Actions	Evaluation
Comfort reestablished during postpartum period.	1. Assess q3–4h for pain. 2. Sitz baths t.i.d. 3. Tucks to epis./hemor. 4. Analgesics as ordered 5. Analgesic spray to epis. 6. Analgesics prior to breast feeding, ½h, p.r.n. 7. Assist changing positions q2h postop. 8. Ice to swollen epis., p.r.n. first 24h. 9. Nipples: no soap, special cleansing, air dry, warm packs for engorgement.	Date: Eval: Signature:
Normal patterns of elimination reestablished by discharge.	1. Enc. vdg. q3–4h. 2. Assess bladder for distention q2–3h until pattern reestab. 3. Enc. fluids to 1500/day. 4. Catheterize p.r.n. 5. Offer stool softener/laxative qh.s. as ordered until BM. 6. Enc. embulation q4h. 7. Enc. fruits/juices t.i.d. 8. Suppository/enema p.r.n. as ordered.	Date: Eval: Signature:
Breastfeeding 10min/breast at each feeding q2–5h by discharge.	1. Assess need for help q fdg. 2. Provide written and verbal instructions at first fdg. 3. Enc. attendance at breastfeeding class. 4. Discuss breast care first postpartum day. 5. Nipple cups for flat/inverted nipples first postpartum day. 6. Enc. rest, fluids, nutrition and analgesics p.r.n.	Date: Eval: Signature:

Prevention of postpartum infection.

1. Enc. mother to use good handwashing prior to breast-feeding.
2. Assess for constriction of milk ducts by tight bra; b.i.d. breast assess.
3. Sitz baths for epis. t.i.d.
4. Assess perineum b.i.d. for signs of infection and report to M.D.
5. Teach wiping from front to back after toileting; clean peri-pad q vdg.; assess for burning on vdg.

Date: _____
Eval: _____

Signature: _____

Knowledge/skills of infant care, self care, contraception, growth and development of infants and parents.

1. Assess knowledge related to: infant care—feeding, handling, transporting, bathing, diapering, taking temperature, signs to call doctor about, checkup, immunizations, mother's self care—bathing, pericare, body changes, contraception, checkup, signs to call doctor about, use of sitz bath.
2. Provide verbal and printed information in each learning need area.
3. Demonstrate and have reinforced practice with mother on skills.
4. Assess support system/desire for public health referral for further learning needs at discharge.

Date: _____
Eval: _____

Signature: _____

Normal uterine involution during postpartum.

1. Assess uterus height, position, firmness, and lochia q15min × 4, q½h × 2, q4h × 24h, b.i.d. thereafter or p.r.n.
2. Enc. vdg. q3–4h; cath. if unable to void and distended with uterine displaced.
3. Massage uterus, express clots p.r.n.
4. Initiate oxytocic as ordered for atony.
5. Inform mother of signs to report indicating atony.

Date: _____
Eval: _____

Signature: _____

121

NURSING CARE PLAN #6
DATA COLLECTION AND ANALYSIS
OUR LADY OF MERCY

Patient Admission Assessment

John T. Fineram age 40
284-6847 7493
Dr. Burns/Snider
Room 231

Date **7-6-86** Informant **Patient**   Disposition of valuables: Safe **none** Relative _____

Time **9 am**   Allergies & Manifestations: Family Doctor **E. J. Burris**

Medicines **none**

Foods **none**   Environmental **none.**

PATIENT HEALTH HISTORY   (Number responses to corresponding category)

1. **Present Illness:**
   Patient's statement of
   reason for admission.
   Onset and progression
   of signs and symptoms.
   What gives relief?
   What aggravates symptoms?

2. **Previous Hospitalizations:**
   Where? Why? When?
   Surgeries

3. **Other Health Problems:**
   What
   Treatment now, past

4. **Medications:**
   Dosages and times
   Taken today
   Brought to hospital
   OTC Drugs

5. **Current Diet:**
   Restrictions/limitations
   Appetite

6. **Limitations:**
   Problems with mobility
   Sensory problems
   Physical (resp., cardiac)
   Activity prior to illness

7. **Sleep:**
   Do you get up at night
   Why? Difficulty, What helps

8. **Menstruation:** Flow
   Last period
   Vaginal discharge

9. **Elimination:**
   Last BM, bowel problems
   Bladder problems

10. **Social History:**
    Marital status, spouse's
    health, occupation,
    living arrangements,
    smoking history, drug/
    alcohol history

① Describes pain in chest as "crushing. It felt as if someone put a vise on my chest. It took my breath away. Am I going to die?" Pain began 45 min p̄ dinner while pt. watching TV. First thought "heartburn" but became ↑ severe. First occurrence. Has brother & father c̄ history of M.I.

② Broken R leg as teenager - skiing accident
③ "I need to lose weight & quit smoking."
④ None
⑤ Good appetite, "Too good - and I love all the wrong things: cheesecake, pastry, steak, eggs."
⑥ Complains of shortness of breath, when walking stairs. "I have no time to exercise and I know I should."
⑦ Sleeps 11 pm - 6 am No problems
⑧ Last BM 7/6 no bowel/bladder problems
⑩ Married, 2 children ages 11, 14
Practicing criminal lawyer - works 55-65 hours per week

Smokes 1½ packs a day, "I've tried to quit but it only makes me nervous." "But now I'll do whatever it takes. This really motivates a person."

"I know the doctor will tell me to cut back on work but I can't live like an invalid - that's no life at all."

"Could you get me a phone? I have a few calls that won't wait."

Courtesy of Our Lady of Mercy Hospital, Mariemont, Ohio.

MIDDLE ADULT: HEART ATTACK

PATIENT ASSESSMENT

Vital Signs: T _98°_ P _120_ R _28_ BP _118/80_ (*H says usual* _146/90_) Apical Pulse _120_

Skin Observations: warm – dry – cyanotic – flushed – jaundiced   Height _6'0"_ Weight _210_
(circle)   other (describe) _pale, diaphoretic, warm_

Level of Consciousness: (X) alert, oriented to person, place, time
(check)   ( ) drowsy, but arouses easily; obeys simple commands
          ( ) stuporous, purposeful response to pain, purposeless response to pain
          ( ) semi-comatose, responds to deep pain
and/or   ( ) coma, no response to deep pain
circle   ( ) anesthetized

Mental/Emotional Status: _Fearful – "Am I going to die?"_

Respiratory Assessment: _Shallow rapid respirations. Lungs clear._

General Observations: Indicate location on diagram

Bleeding   Describe: _no bleeding, rash, decubitis_
Discharge   _Skin intact, + drained, clear_
Rash
Scars
Decubitus

Pain shaded area

Injuries:

Laceration Describe: _none_
Hematoma   _none_
Abrasion   _none_
Burns   _none_

Prosthesis

Dentures: Upper _—_   Contacts _—_
          Lower _—_   Glasses _yes_
Bridgework/Caps _—_   Hearing Aid _—_
Other

Other OBJECTIVE DATA (Additional assessment pertinent to current admission)

\# _Heart sounds clear & regular c̄ occasional premature beat_
\# _Monitor shows normal sinus rhythm with occasional premature_
    ventricular contraction

Safety
✓ Oriented to call system and physical environment
✓ Explained siderail policy
✓ Explained smoking policy
___ Needs assistance with ambulation _(Bed rest)_

Needs
Patient teaching _____
Social Service Referral _____
Admitted by: _M. Knedle_ RN
Primary Nurse _M. Knedle_ RN

Form #4562

NURSING CARE PLAN #6 (Cont.)

Nursing Diagnosis

1. Alteration in comfort: potential for chest pain related to myocardial hypoxia.
2. Potential for complications associated with myocardial hypoxia.

3. Disturbance in self-esteem related to physical limitations.

4. Fear related to MI and possible recurrence.

Goals

1. Patient will verbalize no pain during this 8-h shift. 7/6, 11 P.M.

2. Patient will remain free of complications during hospitalization as evidenced by: stable vital signs, clear heart and lung sounds, normal sinus rhythm.
3. Patient will make two realistic statements regarding ability to safely resume his career. 7/9.
4. Patient will identify high-risk factors in current life-style and measures to minimize their effect. 7/11.

Planned Actions

1. a. Assess patient for pain q1h using verbal and nonverbal cues.
   b. Explain reasons for pain and continued frequent assessment.

   c. Medicate as required.

2. a. Monitor and report any deviation from baseline data: vital signs, lung/heart sounds, sensorium, cardiac rhythm, urine output, skin temperature, daily weight.
   b. Apply antiembolism stockings.

3. a. Assess patient cognitive/affective level of understanding of MI via reflection and open-ended questions.

Rationale

1. a. Pain is indicator of myocardial hypoxia. Pain indicates unmet O_2 need.
   b. Beginning at learner's level of understanding facilitates learning. Understanding rationale enhances patient cooperation in procedures.
   c. (1) Pain increases O_2 demands.
      (2) Determine effect of med.

2. a. Assessment data for indication of physical deterioration.

   b. Aids circulation of venous blood and decreases potential for venostasis.
3. a. Teaching begins at patient's level of understanding.

MIDDLE ADULT: HEART ATTACK

Planned Actions

    b. Clarify the prognosis and information given by M.D.

    c. Discuss concept patient has of self as "invalid."

    d. Reinforce patient's own problem-solving skills in dealing with situation.

4 **a.** Approach: nonjudgmental.

    b. Assess patient knowledge of heart disease and contributing factors.

    c. Provide information and clarificiation.

    d. Using open-ended question, help patient recognize factors in own life.

    e. Using open-ended questions, help patient begin problem solving to reduce risk factors.

    f. Plan family conference when physical status permits to discuss life-style alterations.

Rationale

    b. Patient may have decreased perception under stress.

    c. MI patients can gradually resume work status with varied alterations.

    d. Self-esteem need.

4. **a.** Minimize guilt feelings.

    b. Teaching begins at learner's level of understanding.

    c. Improve patient knowledge base for problem solving.

    d.e.f. Participation in developing health care plan enhances cooperation and restores control to individual. Involvement of family will support necessary changes.

NURSING CARE PLAN #6 (Cont.)

Evaluation

1. Goal met. "I haven't had any pain all evening."
   7/6 _____ *M Knedle, R.N.*

2. Goal met. Patient remains free of complications during hospitalization.
   7/16 _____ *M. knedle R.N.*

3. Goal met. Patient states, "Maybe I can hire a research assistant to lighten my work." "I'll limit my case load."
   7/9 _____ *M. Knedle R.N.*

4. Goal partially met. Recognizes: weight factor, high BP, smoking, lack of exercise, overwork, family history. States, "I need to smoke. It helps me think. I can't quit cold turkey." Agrees to weight reduction diet.
   7/11 _____ *M. Knedle R.N.*

Review of Nursing Process/ Care Plan

1. Continue goal and actions.

4. New Data:
   "I need to smoke. It helps me think. I can't quit cold turkey." New short-term goal: Patient will decrease smoking to one pack/day for 2 wk and consider progressive reduction. 7/25
   New Actions:
   1. Check progress qd.
   2. Reinforce decreased smoking.
   3. Encourage family support.

NURSING CARE PLAN #7
DATA COLLECTION AND ANALYSIS

SENIOR ADULT:
DEPRESSION

FLOOR _1W_   NURSES ADMISSION ASSESSMENT   ROOM NUMBER _108_

NAME _Fred Morgan / 78 years_   ALLERGIES (Write in RED) _none_

Name Preferred _Fred_

Admission Date _2-1-86_   Admission Time _2 PM_   Male (X)   Female ( )

Admitting Diagnosis _unable to do own ADL_

Vital Signs: B/P _126/80_   Temp _97⁶_   Pulse _88_   Resp. _18_   Height _6'1"_ Weight _160_

Pacemaker: Type _none_   Set Rate_____   Demand_____

Head: Hair and Scalp Condition: dry___ oily _X_ abrasions___ lumps___ scars___

Neck: Abrasions _Ō_ Bruises _Ū_ Reddened areas _Ō_ Lumps _Ō_ Scars _Ō_

Eyes: Normal Appearance _X_ Reddened _Ō_ Swollen _Ō_ Prosthesis _Ū_ Drainage _Ō_

Nose: Normal Appearance _X_ Swollen___ Deviated___ Drainage___ Hair___

Ears: Normal Appearance _X_ Swollen___ Deformed___ Drainage___ Hair___ Wax___

Condition of Mouth: Color of Gums _PINK_   Open Sores _Ō_ Laceration _Ō_

Condition of Lips: Color _PINK_ Dry _X_ Sores___ Scars___ Deformed___

Teeth: Natual___ Decayed___ Dentures _X_ : upper _X_ : lower _Ō_ Broken or Chipped _no_

Tongue: Normal Appearance _X_ Color_____ Swollen___ Lacerated___ Deformed___

Courtesy Meadowbrook Care Center, Cincinnati, Ohio.

NURSING CARE PLAN #7
DATA COLLECTION AND ANALYSIS (Cont.)

NAME _Fred Morgan_   NURSES ADMISSION ASSESSMENT - PAGE 2   Room Number _____

HEAD: REMARKS _Normal (unshaven)_

ARMS AND HANDS: Skin Condition: dry _X_ oily___ Condition of Nails: _yellowed, dirty_

    Edema___ Scars___ Contractures___ Bruises___ Rash___ Decubiti___ Deformity_____

    Reddened Areas___ Abrasions___ Cold___ Warm___ Mottled___ Prosthesis___ Surgical Site_____

    Amputation_____ REMARKS: _____

TRUNK: Skin condition: dry _X_ oily___

    Back: Scars___ Bruises___ Rash___ Decubiti___ Reddened Area___ Abrasions___ Lumps___

        Deformity___ Surgical Site___ REMARKS: _Skin "hangs" - no turgor_

    Front: Scars___ Bruises___ Rash___ Decubiti___ Reddened Area___ Abrasions___ Lumps___

        Obese___ Deformity___ Surgical Site___ REMARKS: _Appears gaunt, thin_

GENITILIA: Condition of skin: dry _X_ oily___ Edema___ Scars___ Rash___ Abrasions___

    Decubiti___ Reddened Area___ Surgical Site___ Lumps___ Drainage___ Colostomy_____

    REMARKS: _____

BOWEL & BLADDER: Continent _X_ Incontinent: Bowel___ : Bladder___ Catheter___ : Type_____

    Bowel & Bladder Training___ Recurrent Infections___ Diaper___ Special Peri-Care_____

    Special Anal Care___ Chronic constipation___ Uses Fracture Pan_____

    REMARKS: _____

LEGS & FEET: Skin condition: dry _X_ oily___ Condition of Nails: _____

    Edema___ Scars___ Contractures___ Bruises___ Rash___ Decubiti___ Deformity_____

    Reddened Area___ Abrasions___ Cold___ Warm___ Mottled___ Prosthesis___

    Surgical Site___ Amputation___ REMARKS: _____

FIVE SENSES: Hearing: No problems _✓_ Impaired___ Hearing Aid___ Deaf___ Wax___ Drainage___

    Sight: No problems___ Glasses _X_ Impaired Vision___ Blind___ Prosthesis_____

    Speech: No problems _✓_ Aphasic___ Mumbles___ Stutter___ Lisp___ Mute___

        Language Spoken _Note: responds only to direct questions_

    Touch: No problems _✓_ Impaired___

    Smell: No problems _✓_ Impaired___ REMARKS: _____

SENIOR ADULT: DEPRESSION

NAME _Fred Morgan_   NURSES ADMISSION ASSESSMENT – PAGE 3   Room Number _108_

HABITS: Appetite _Poor_   Feeds Self _✓_   Requires Feeding _____   Snacks _____

     Fluid Intake _____   Retires Early _✓_   Naps _✓_   Sleeping Medication _Dalmane_

                                         Awakens 2-3x per night   _15 mg "0"_

     Hobbies, Interests, Likes, Dislikes _retired carpenter_

     REMARKS: _"Food just doesn't taste good anymore."_

AMBULATION: Ambulatory _X_ : Independent _X_   assist needed ___   walker ___   cane ___   wheelchair ___

              Transfer Only ___   Bedridden ___

              REMARKS: _____

NURSE'S ADMISSION NOTES:

     Means of transportation to this facility: _Car accompanied by son_

     Name of transporting agency (If applicable): _NA_

     Did someone accompany the resident and if so whom? _____

     Resident transferred from: _NA_

     Attending Physician: _C. R. Roth_

     Was the Attending Physician notified of the resident's arrival? _yes_

     Was the resident accompanied by all necessary transfer information? _NA_

     Were the Doctor's Orders confirmed? _yes_

     What was the resident's reaction to admission? _"I'm tired, just let me rest."_

     Was the resident oriented to the floor plan of the Nursing Unit? _yes_

     Did the resident have any specific requests upon admission? _no_

     SUMMARY REVIEW: _Son states father is depressed and withdrawn._
     Does not eat, no interest in any activity, was not
     bathing, shaving or doing personal hygiene.

                                                 Date of Admission Assessment _2-1-86_

                                                 Time: _4 PM_

         Plan of Care? Yes _✓_ No ___

Signature of the Nurse doing the Assessment: _J. Olson, RN_

NURSING CARE PLAN #7
DATA COLLECTION AND ANALYSIS (Cont.)

SOCIAL HISTORY

MEADOWBROOK CARE CENTER

RESIDENT'S NAME: _Fred Morgan_

DATE OF ADMISSION: _2-1-86_

MEDICAL DIAGNOSIS AND PRESENT LEVEL OF FUNCTIONING, (PHYSICAL AND MENTAL):

"No physical complaints; I'm not interested in anything - just leave me alone & let me rest." (No facial expression or eye contact) "I'm no good to anyone - I can't do a thing." Denies feeling suicidal "I wouldn't do that."

FORMER LIVING ARRANGEMENTS, REASONS FOR ADMISSION AND INTENDED LENGTH OF STAY:

Son lives out of town. Mr. Morgan unable to perform ADL's - not eating. Weight loss of 11 lbs in two months.
Rarely went out of house except for church.
May be able to return home if able to do self-care

RESIDENT'S AWARENESS OF DIAGNOSIS AND ATTITUDES TOWARD AGING AND DEATH:

Wife died 1 year ago, "I can't understand why she had to die. I wish it had been me. It's hard to be the one left."
"I want to be with her again."

RESIDENT'S AND FAMILY'S REACTIONS TOWARD ADMISSION: _States, "I liked my own house. When you live in a place 30 years, it's hard to move." Mr. Fred Morgan states "My son is busy with his own life. He doesn't have time for me."_

FAMILY'S SUGGESTIONS TO FACILITATE ADJUSTMENT TO MEADOWBROOK CARE CENTER:

Son: "Dad needs to put on weight. He'd feel better if he was eating better. He needs friends ... something to do."

SENIOR ADULT: DEPRESSION

SOCIAL HISTORY
PAGE TWO

FAMILY NETWORK AND IMPORTANT DYNAMICS: _Son (only child) lives_
out of town - two grandchildren

EDUCATION AND WORK HISTORY, ATTITUDE TOWARD RETIREMENT: _____

Enjoyed retirement, until wife died. Was a carpenter -
retired at 65 years old in excellent health.

SPECIAL RESPONSIBILITIES, ACTIVITIES, OR TALENTS: _Was active in_
Church work with wife. Has not attended in
past 6 months despite repeated contacts from
group

T. Olson, RN
SIGNATURE

_2-1-86_
DATE

NURSING CARE PLAN #7 (Cont.)

Nursing Diagnosis

1. Alteration in nutrition: less than body requirements associated with lack of interest in food.

2. Social isolation associated with unresolved losses.

3. Disturbance in self-esteem related to feelings of worthlessness

4. Potential for violence: self-directed related to feelings of depression.

Goals

1. Short-term: Client will gain 1 lb by the end of the week. 1/8
   Long-term: Client's weight will stabilize @ his preadmission level within 3 mo. 5/1

2. Short-term: Client will participate in one new activity by Wednesday, 1/10.
   Long-term: Client will initiate contact c̄ another resident @ a time other than meals or planned group activities, within 1 mo. 3/1

3. Short-term: Client will make one positive statement of self-worth within 48 hr. 2/3

4. Client will deny suicidal plans or ideation throughout stay in nursing home. Evaluate Fridays of each wk.

Planned Actions

1. a. Observe, record, and report I & O.
   b. Weigh q A.M.
   c. Assess food preferences.

   d. Assist client in filling out daily menu.

   e. Consult with physician and dietitian regarding between-meal snacks, high calorie and high protein food supplements, possible vitamin supplements.
   f. Assist client with hygiene before meals.
   g. Encourage client to sit with others in the dining room @ mealtimes.

Rationale

1. a.b. Monitor client's progress/ evaluate effectiveness of plan.
   c. Taking into account client's likes/dislikes may stimulate appetite.
   d. Involve client in plan to increase cooperation. Ensure nutritionally balanced meal.
   e. Meet nutritional needs of client.

   f. Increase psychological and physical readiness to eat.
   g. Normal eating situation tends to stimulate appetite.

SENIOR ADULT: DEPRESSION

Planned Interventions	*Rationale*
2. a. Assess the existence, extent and impact of unresolved losses through use of open-ended and direct questions.	**2. a.** Must assess types of unresolved losses and importance to client in order to fully implement plan (Note: elderly frequently have multiple unresolved losses).
b. Encourage client to verbalize feelings regarding losses. **c.** Share own observations of client's behavior and seek clarification/confirmation.	**b.c.** Increase database; assist client in developing an awareness of predominant feelings.
d. Spend 10 min sitting c̄ client b.i.d.; use touch as appropriate; remain c̄ client despite lack of ability to verbalize.	**d.** Build rapport, develop trust. Convey unconditional acceptance so client is free to express feelings.
e. Look over the daily activity calendar c̄ the client and leave a copy in his room; specifically suggest choosing one activity.	**e.** Involve client to improve cooperation. Individualize plan to insure its likelihood of success. Decrease isolation.
f. Encourage client to sit c̄ others in the dining room @ meal times. **g.** Introduce client to other residents on the unit.	**f.g.** Gradually "repeople" client's life-supply opportunities for development of meaningful interpersonal relationships s̄ overwhelming him. Reinforce sense of belonging.
3. a. Assess client's interests through use of open-ended and direct questions.	**3. a.** Necessary data to guide plan.
b. Encourage patient to verbalize about himself, especially his present feelings.	**b.** Continue assessment. Convey acceptance of client. Increase client awareness of feelings.
c. Continue nursing actions 2.c. and 2.d.	**c.** Same as 2.c. and 2.d.
d. Maximize choices client can make. **e.** Assist c̄ grooming as needed. **f.** Give merited praise and recognition based on specific, accurate observation.	**d.e.f.** Rebuild self-esteem.

NURSING CARE PLAN #7 (Cont.)

Planned Actions

4. **a.** Be direct in asking client if he is presently suicidal.
   b. Make verbal agreement c̄ client that he will notify nursing staff if feeling out of control or suicidal.
   c. Move client to room closer to nurse's station if feeling suicidal.
   d. Increase frequency of room checks.

   e. Monitor client behavior; observe especially for changes in mood/or levels of energy (be aware of greater risk following these changes).
   f. Alert all staff regarding client's suicidal potential.
   g. Continue nursing action 4. from b.
   h. Permit verbalization of suicidal feelings, do not ignore them or argue c̄ client about them.
   i. Carefully document client behavior and nursing actions.

Rationale

4. **a.** Determine immediate goal for intervention.
   b. Involve client in plan to ensure its success.

   c. Increase nurse's accessibility to client and increase opportunities for observation.
   d. Prevent, interfere with, or interrupt any self-destructive behavior.
   e. Provide data c̄ which to evaluate suicide potential; changes may signal increased suicide risk.

   f. Provide safety and security for client.
   g. Same as 4.b.

   h. Establish trust. Recognize importance of intent.

   i. Ensure consistency of care.

SENIOR ADULT: DEPRESSION

Review of Nursing Process/
Care Plan

Evaluation

1. Goal not met. Client's weight remained the same.
   1/8_____ *F. Olson, RN*

2. Goal met. Client attended the Tuesday evening Bible study group, though the group leader said client did not contribute to the discussion.
   1/10____ *F. Olson, RN*

1. Continue goal and actions; change evaluation date for short-term goal to 1/16.
   New Data:
   > After first refusing to eat more than desserts and coffee, client finished entire meal following brief explanation by nurse of the importance of a balanced diet for good nutrition.

   New Action:
   1. Reinforce importance of balanced diet with brief explanation.

2. New Data:
   > Client states regarding wife's death: "You know, I still feel kind of stunned . . . it doesn't seem real yet . . . I mean, how can I face other people without her?"

   New Nursing Diagnosis:
   > Social withdrawal related to delayed grief reaction over loss of wife.

   New Short-term Goal:
   > Client will verbalize feelings of sorrow caused by the loss of his wife within 1 wk. 2/17

   New Action:
   1. Assist client to review his relationship $\bar{c}$ his wife, including shared pleasures and regrets, through use of reflection and open-ended questions.

NURSING CARE PLAN #7 (Cont.)

Evaluation

3. Goal met. Client states "I used
   to be a pretty good carpenter
   . . . I've always been good @
   working with my hands."

   2/3 _*J. Olson, RN*_

4. Goal met. Client agreed to seek
   out staff if feeling suicidal or out
   of control, though he continues
   to deny feeling suicidal.

   2/7 _*J. Olson, RN.*_

Review of Nursing Process/
Care Plan

3. New Data:
   Client states regarding loss of
      work role: "I still can't get
      used to being so useless . . .
      you know p̄ my wife died I sold
      the house and had to give up
      my workshop and all my
      woodworking tools . . . I used
      to work all day on my proj-
      ects; still would if I had my
      tools."
   New Short-term Goal:
      Client will begin woodworking
      project in OT by 2/7.
   New Actions:
      1. Consult with occupational
         therapist regarding wood-
         working projects for client.
      2. Discuss working in OT c̄
         client and set up a schedule
         c̄ him.
      3. Reassess and evaluate client
         self-esteem using direct
         questions.

4. Maintain plan.

Index